CANCER ETIOLOGY, DIAGNOSIS AND TREATMENTS

ENDOMETRIAL CANCER

A COMPREHENSIVE CLINICAL AND TRANSLATIONAL UPDATE

CANCER ETIOLOGY, DIAGNOSIS AND TREATMENTS

Additional books in this series can be found on Nova's website under the Series tab.

Additional e-books in this series can be found on Nova's website under the e-book tab.

CANCER ETIOLOGY, DIAGNOSIS AND TREATMENTS

ENDOMETRIAL CANCER

A COMPREHENSIVE CLINICAL AND TRANSLATIONAL UPDATE

IVAN DIAZ-PADILLA
AND
JESUS GARCIA-DONAS
EDITORS

New York

For permission to use material from this book please contact us:
Telephone 631-231-7269; Fax 631-231-8175
Web Site: http://www.novapublishers.com

Library of Congress Cataloging-in-Publication Data

ISBN: 978-1-63321-323-4

Library of Congress Control Number: 2014942815

Published by Nova Science Publishers, Inc. † New York

Contents

In: Endometrial Cancer
Editors: I. Diaz-Padilla, J. Garcia-Donas
ISBN: 978-1-63321-323-4

Chapter I

The Epidemiology of Endometrial Cancer

Stephanie Irene Ayre and Laurie Elit*
Department of Obstetrics and Gynecology,
McMaster University, Hamilton, Canada

Abstract

Endometrial cancer is the most common reproductive cancer in women in developed countries and the fourth most common cancer overall. The cumulative risk in more developed countries is 1.58%, compared to a cumulative risk of 0.67% in less developed regions. Many epidemiologic studies have been performed to determine the risk factors for endometrial cancer and the degree to which they influence incidence and mortality. Through a thorough search of the literature we aimed to establish and review the current literature related to endometrial cancer risk as well as evaluate the newer methods for prevention and lifestyle modification.

Studies have shown increased incidence of disease in women who carry certain genetic mutations like in Lynch syndrome (MSH2, MLH1, MSH6, PMS2), while exposure to unopposed estrogen is believed to

* Corresponding author: Laurie Elit, 699 Concession Street, Hamilton, Ontario, Canada L8V 5C2. Phone: 905 3895688. Fax: 905 575-634. E-mail: laurie.elit@jcc.hhsc.ca.

account for increased rates in women with infertility, exposure to certain hormones, obesity, diabetes and polycystic ovary syndrome.

Factors that appear to be protective include oral contraception use, IUDs, physical activity, smoking, and immune conditions like systemic lupus erythematous.

There is significant data supporting several well-known endometrial cancer risk factors including age, race, obesity and unopposed estrogen use. Epidemiologic studies help researchers focus their questions on biologic mechanisms for disease which could be exploited in either treatment (progesterone use for women with grade 1 metastatic endometrial cancer) or prevention (progesterone use in women with endometrial hyperplasia). The role of diet, exercise and agents like metformin in preventing endometrial cancer or survivorship after being diagnosed with disease continues to require further evaluation.

Keywords: Risk factors for endometrial cancer, epidemiology for endometrial cancer, Lynch syndrome, unopposed estrogen, obesity, infertility

Introduction

Endometrial cancer is the most common reproductive cancer in women in developed countries and the fourth most common cancer overall. The cumulative risk in more developed countries, according to Globocan 2008, is 1.58%, compared to a cumulative risk of 0.67% in less developed regions. Rates are highest in North America and Central and Eastern Europe and lowest in Western and Middle Africa and South-Central Asia [1]. More recent data from the National Cancer Institute in the United States shows an increasing incidence for United States citizens. Based on SEER data from 2008-2010 it is estimated that 2.69% or 1/37 women born today will be diagnosed with uterine cancer at some point during their lifetime [2].

Data from the United States also shows significant discrepancies between races. White women have a higher incidence of disease when compared to all other ethnicities; however Black women are shown to have much higher rates of mortality. From 2006 to 2010 the incidence rates for White women were estimated at 25.1 per 100,000 women. This is compared to 22.2 for Black women, 18.6 for Asian/Pacific Islander, 20.3 for American Indian/Alaska Native and 19.4 for Hispanic women. Mortality rates for Black women were 7.4 per 100,000 women compared to4.0 for White women, 2.6 for Asian/Pacific Islander, 3.2 for American Indian/Alaska native and 3.3 for

Hispanic women [2]. It is not clear if there is a genetic predisposition for black women to with endometrial cancer to have a poorer prognosis or if this is related to other factors such as access to care and the quality of care they receive.

On a global scale, incidence rates of endometrial cancer are highest in the 70-74 age group, followed by 65-69 years of age. Mortality, however, is highest for those greater than 75 years of age [1]. Comparatively, American data from 2006-2010 showed that the median age at diagnosis was 62 years of age with 33.4% of patients diagnosed between 55-64 years of age. In this data set 26.9 % died between the ages of 65-74 [2]. It is not clear if women in high resource settings have their endometrial cancer identified at an earlier age due to better access to health care and diagnostic techniques (i.e., transvaginal ultrasound and endometrial aspiration), or if there is some other explanation for the earlier age of diagnosis.

When discussing the epidemiology of endometrial cancer it is important to acknowledge the vast heterogeneity within this cancer. The broader category of endometrial cancer, or 'cancer of the uterine corpus' may include both type I and type II endometrial cancers. Type I or 'endometrioid type' accounts for approximately 80% of endo-metrial cancers, while type II or 'non-endometrioid' accounts for 20% and includes adenosquamous, serous papillary, clear cell and undifferentiated types [3]. While it was previously believed that the two types were distinctly different entities, there is emerging evidence that type I and type II may have more similar epidemiologic risk factors than previously thought. Setiawan et al. published data from 10 cohort studies and 14 case-control studies in 2013. The data included 14,069 endometrial cancer cases and 35,312 controls from the United States, Canada, Europe, Australia and China. They found that parity, OCP use, cigarette smoking, age at menarche and diabetes were associated with type I and type II tumors to a similar extent. While they did find that BMI had a great effect on type I tumors, they also showed a positive association with type II tumors with an odds ratio of 1.12 (95% CI 1.09 – 1.14) [4].

The GOG recently addressed this question through GOG 210 [5]. Here a central pathology review standardized the tumor histologies and grade. They found in 2244 type I cancers and 581 type II cancers that those with type II cancers were more likely to be older, non-white, multiparous, current smokers and less often obese. Grade 3 endometrioid cancers had a profile more in keeping with women in the type II cancer category. The grade 3 endometrial cancer group more often had histories of breast cancer without tamoxifen exposure compared to the other type II cases who more likely had breast cancer with tamoxifen exposure. Yang et al. in a study of 114,409 women in the National Institutes of Health AARP Diet and Health Study (1995-2006) also reported a strong relationship of type II tumors with black versus white (RR 2.18 vs 0.66, p (hetero-geneity)=0.0004) and having a family history of breast cancer (RR 1.93 vs 0.80, p(heterogeneity)=0.002) [6].

Despite emerging evidence from these newer studies the majority of previous studies in the literature focus on type I endometrial cancer. In this type, factors which increase the amount of unopposed estrogen in the circulatory system are believed to increase the risk of developing hyperplasia and cancer. These include obesity, anovulatory cycles, as seen in PCOS, and estrogen-replacement therapy.

Alternatively, factors which inhibit production of estrogen are believed to decrease the risk including cigarette smoking, alcohol consumption and progesterone-containing intrauterine devices [7].

Table 1. Risk factors for Endometrial Cancer

Risk Factors	Impact on Risk
Age (Increased)	↑
White race	↑
Residence in North America and Northern Europe	↑
Lynch syndrome	↑
BRCA 1/ BRCA 2	↑
Nulliparity	↑
Infertility	↑
Early menarche	↑
Late menopause	↑
OCP use	↓
IUD use	↓
Unopposed Estrogen use	↑
Tamoxifen use	↑
Obesity	↑
Physical Activity	↓
Diet	↔
Alcohol consumption	↔
Smoking	↓
Systemic Lupus Erythematous	↓
Polycystic Ovarian Syndrome	↑
Diabetes	↑

↑ increased risk.
↓ decreased risk.
↔ no clear increase or decrease in risk.

Genetic Factors

Most endometrial cancers are thought to be sporadic but a small number do have a hereditary basis. The two most common associations are with Lynch syndrome and BRCA 1 and BRCA 2.

Lynch Syndrome

Lynch syndrome otherwise known as hereditary nonpolyposis colorectal cancer (HNPCC) is an autosomally dominant cancer susceptibility syndrome associated with early onset cancers of the colon, rectum, ovary, small bowel, ureter, renal pelvis and/or endometrium.

Of all women with endometrial cancer, 2.5% of them have Lynch syndrome [8-12]. Of women with endometrial cancer younger than 50 years old, approximately 10% have Lynch syndrome. The life time risk of someone with Lynch syndrome developing endometrial cancer is 40-60%. This rate is similar to the rate of women with Lynch syndrome developing colorectal cancer [13-17]. In fact, of all women with Lynch syndrome, half will develop endometrial cancer first and colorectal cancer later while the remainder develop colorectal cancer first and later endometrial cancer. A small number of women will have both cancers at the time of diagnosis. The life time risk of a person with Lynch syndrome developing ovarian cancer is 10-12%.

Lynch syndrome is due to a germ-line mutation of one of the DNA mismatch repair genes hMSH2, hMLH1, hMSH6, or hPMS2. In Lynch syndrome, one non-functional allele is inherited. When there is loss of the corresponding allele, repair of the genetic DNA is defective in the target tissue. hMLH1 and hMSH2 account for over 90% of the diagnosed Lynch syndrome cases.

The lifetime risk of endometrial cancer does vary based on the mutation for example, hMSH2 is 40%-61% [15, 16, 18], hMLH1 27-42% [15, 16], and hMSH6 71% [16]. This is compared to the population risk of endometrial cancer of 3% or the risk in women tested and found not to have the mutation which is 8% [19].

Immunohistochemical or microsatellite instability testing can be performed on paraffin embedded tissue as an intermediate step prior to performing germline mutational analysis. There appears to be limited efficacy for screening high risk women with serial ultrasound [20, 21] or endometrial biopsy [22]. There is currently an ongoing multi-institutional study comparing levonorgesterel oral contraceptive pill versus depmedroxyprogesterone acetate

[23]. Risk reducing surgery with prophylactic hysterectomy and bilateral salpingo-oophorectomy (BSO) has been shown to minimize the occurrence of gynecologic malignancy in women with Lynch syndrome. A prospective cohort study of 315 women with germ-line mutation associated with Lynch syndrome were followed [23]. Sixty-one women had a prophylactic hysterectomy and 47 had a prophylactic BSO. When age-matched to mutation positive women without prophylactic surgery, there were 69 women who developed endometrial cancer in the control group for an incidence density of 0.045 per woman year compared to zero in the prophylactic surgery group ($p<0.001$).

Median age of endometrial cancer was 46 years (range 30-69 years). As well, ovarian cancer was diagnosed in 12 women in the control group for an incidence density of 0.005 per woman-year compared to zero in the prophylactic surgery group ($p=0.09$).

There has been one case report of a primary peritoneal cancer in a 56 year old woman who had Lynch syndrome and had a prophylactic BSO at age 44 years old [24].

BRCA 1 and BRCA 2

There appears to be mixed reviews on the relationship of BRCA 1 and BRCA 2 in the occurrence of endometrial cancer. Hornreich presented a case report of sisters with the same BRCA 1 mutation who also developed serous uterine cancer [25]. Levine et al. reviewed 199 Ashkenzi Jewish women with endometrial cancer from a single institution and 3 out of 199 had a founder BRCA 1 or BRCA 2 germ line mutation [26]. This rate is in keeping with that of the Ashkenazi population (2%). Goshen reported on 56 women with uterine serous papillary cancer in Ontario, Canada and none of them had a BRCA 1 or BRCA 2 mutation [27]. Beiner et al. conducted a prospective study of 857 women with BRCA 1 or BRCA 2 carriers ages 45-70 year old. During the 3.3 years of follow-up, 6 developed endometrial cancer. Four of them had been exposed to tamoxifen. Compared to those who had not used tamoxifen, the BRCA carriers did not have a different rate of endometrial cancer compared to the general population [28]. Beiner's study reflects some of the difficulties when addressing the relationship of BRCA 1 and BRCA2 with uterine cancer. There can be confounding with use of agents such as tamoxifen for breast cancer as this is the population in whom we are most likely to know the BRCA 1 and BRCA 2 status.

Reproductive Factors

Nulliparity and Infertility

Exposure of the endometrium to 'unopposed estrogen' is a well known cause of endometrial hyperplasia and cancer. Pregnancy causes significant changes in endogenous estrogen and progesterone levels and it has been suggested that pregnancy reduces the amount of time that the endometrium is exposed to unopposed estrogen [29]. The literature supports a significant association between nulliparity and elevated endometrial cancer risk, while increasing number of births has been shown to reduce risk.

On average, studies have shown a 2-5 times increased risk of endometrial cancer in nulliparous women [29, 30].

Several studies have looked at this association and hypothesized the possible causes. A large prospective cohort study in Norway followed 765,756 women for an average of 12.2 years until December 31, 1991. The study showed an incidence rate ratio (IRR) of endometrial cancer for nulliparous women ages 30-44 of 3.09 (95% CI 1.93-4.95). Women ages 45-56 had an IRR Of 1.41 (0.97-2.05). The reduction in risk with first pregnancy was more pronounced than that observed for subsequent pregnancies.

Furthermore, increasing time since last birth was related to an increased risk of endometrial cancer. On average, the risk increased by 20% per 5 year time interval since last birth (IRR 1.20; 95% CI 1.08-1.34) [29]. It is thought that this association may be secondary to mechanical shed of malignant or pre-malignant epithelial cells at each delivery.

Therefore, a later age at delivery, as well as multiple deliveries, decreases the amount of time which these cells have to proliferate.

This has been reinforced by several more recent studies. Bevier et al. published a study in 2010 in which they analyzed reproductive factors influencing endometrial and ovarian cancer rates in 5.7 million women selected from the Swedish-Family Cancer databases. They showed a relative risk (RR) of 0.47 (95% CI 0.42-0.52) for those patients with one child compared to nulliparous women. Women with 3-4 children had a RR of 0.36 (95% CI 0.32-0.40) and those with more than 10 children had a RR of 0.25 (0.10-0.58). In patients who had only one child the RR for those ages 30-39 was 0.75 (0.68-0.83) while those over 40 years of age had a RR of 0.51 (0.44-0.58) [30]. Other studies have reinforced this data and also found that the protective association was similar for both type I and type II endometrial cancers and was not influenced by BMI or exogenous hormone use. They also showed that a longer period between births decreases the risk of endometrial cancer. The evidence is mixed in terms of whether this data is specific to full-term live births or all pregnancies regardless of outcomes. Some studies have shown that the above associations are also displayed among those women who have had terminations or miscarriages, while other studies have shown that their rates are the same as nulliparous women [31-33].

Studies have also suggested that there may be an independent association between infertility and endometrial cancer outside of the risks associated with nulliparity. This may be secondary to anovulation and elevated androgens, as seen in patients with polycystic ovarian syndrome, as well as a lack of monthly sloughing of the lining noted in oligomenorrhea [34].

Althius et al. published a retrospective cohort study in 2005 of 8,431 US women evaluated for infertility from 1965-1988.

The study showed a standar-dized incidence rate for endometrial cancer of 1.56 (95% CI 1.1-2.1) for women with a history of infertility [35].

The question also arises as to whether infertility treatments cause an increase in endometrial cancer rates later in life. Of particular interest is the use of the pharmacologic agent clomiphene citrate.

This frequently used infertility treatment is a selective estrogen receptor modulator, with a similar structure to tamoxifen; a drug which has also been linked with endometrial cancer risk. The above study published by Althius et al. in 2005 found that clomiphene may increase uterine cancer risk RR 1.79 (95% CI 0.9-3.4) and this may be increased with increasing dose, number of cycles used and time elapsed since initial use [35].

A retrospective cohort study of 12,193 US women published in 2013 by Brinton et al. has re-evaluated the association between fertility treatments and endometrial cancer. They did not find statistical significance for most associations between fertility drugs and endometrial cancer. In their study clomiphene was shown to have a hazards ratio of 1.39 (95% CI 0.96-2.01).

This association remained unchanged when adjusted for number of births, age at menarche, BMI at age 40 or cause of infertility. They did not illustrate trends associated with increasing cumulative doses or with the number of cycles used. They did however show that patients who received clomiphene prior to age 30 were at increased risk (HR 1.95; 95% CI 1.24-3.00).

Those who used gonadotropins in the study were also at a non-significantly increased risk of endometrial cancer (HR 1.34; 95% CI 0.76-2.37). The authors of the article emphasize limitations of the study including smaller sample sizes and the fact that patients studied were still young and had not yet reached the peak age for endometrial cancer incidence [36].

Menstrual Factors

The impact of unopposed estrogens is also believed to be central to the association seen with early menarche and late menopause. Several studies have shown a significant increase in risk of endometrial cancer in those women who are believed to have a longer reproductive life. In 2009, Dossus et al. examined data from the European Prospective Investigation into Cancer and Nutrition (EPIC) study. Among 302,618 women who were eligible for the study; 1,012 incident cases of endometrial cancer were found.

Results of the study showed risk reductions of 7-8% for each additional year of menstrual life. The study found that endometrial cancer was lower among women with a later age at menarche (HR 0.72; 95% CI 0.58-0.90) when comparing women with menarche at age 15 to menarche before age 12. They also found that women with late menopause after age 55 compared to prior to age 50 had a higher risk of endometrial cancer (HR 2.20; 95% CI 1.61-3.01). Subgroup analyses showed that these rates remained the same when analyzed for variables by country, age at cancer diagnosis, menopausal status at baseline or obesity [32].

Contraception

The study performed by Dossus also found an association between oral contraception (OC) use and decreased risks of endometrial cancer. Similar to a prolonged reproductive life, they found that the risk of endometrial cancer decreased by 7-8% for each year of OC used. Results of the study showed that compared to non-users, users of OC were at a reduced risk of developing endometrial cancer (HR 0.65; 95% CI 0.56-0.75) and among users duration of use was inversely associated with risk (HR for >10 years 0.58; 95% CI 0.42-0.79) compared to users for one year or less. While the study indicates that OC use included some form of progesterone it is less clear how many patients were on combined versus progestin only preparations and the dosages of each. The association with OC use and decreased risks can be explained in part by the suppression of menstrual cycles. According to Dossus, during the follicular phase of the menstrual cycle (of women not taking OC), the release of estrogen alone increases endometrial mitotic activity. Women taking OCs are gene-rally exposed to a combined preparation and thus receive both estrogen and progesterone to counteract the estrogen activity, as well, lower postmenopausal endogenous estrogen concentrations have been observed in past OC users [32]. Multiple studies have supported the above results and also shown a difference based on the amount of progesterone in the preparation and the BMI of the patient [37-39]. A case control study performed by Maxwell in 2006 examined 434 endometrial cancer cases and 2557 controls identified from the Cancer and Steroid Hormone (CASH) study in the United States. The study showed that both high potency progestins (OR 0.21 95% CI 0.10-0.43) and low potency progestins (0.39; 95% CI0.25-0.60) were protective against developing endometrial cancer. They also showed that high potency progestins provided significantly more protection than low potency when accounting for BMI. Among women with a BMI of 22.1 kg/m^2 or higher progestins conferred a significantly lower risk of endometrial cancer than those who used low potency (OR 0.31; 95% CI 0.11-0.92) while those with a BMI less than 22.1 kg/m^2 did not show this association (OR 1.36; 95% CI 0.39-4.70) [37].

More recently interest has been focused on the potential benefits of progesterone containing intrauterine devices. Many studies have looked into the possible effects of non-hormonal IUDs and most have found a decreased risk of endometrial cancer in those patients treated with non-hormonal IUDs. A meta-analysis of 10 case control studies from 1966-2007 found an almost 50% reduction in endometrial cancer risk with non-hormonal IUD use. (Pooled OR 0.54; 95% CI 0.47-0.63). The mechanism of action is still not fully understood but it is thought that IUDs may cause an alteration in the endometrial lining secondary to a state of chronic inflammation. Molecular studies have also been performed to examine the associations with progestin-implanted IUDs. It is believed that tumor suppressor genes may play a large role in the etiology of endometrial cancer.

A study published by Orbo et al. in 2006 evaluated the PTEN tumor suppressor gene, a gene which when inactivated is believed to be one of the earliest steps in endometrial carcinogenesis.

In the study, they examined cohorts treated with progestin-implanted IUDs, cyclic oral progestins and surveillance only. All groups went through pre- and post-treatment endometrial biopsies. All groups had similar proportions of latent precursors at intake but the IUD group had the highest rate of regression with 62% pretherapy and 5% post-therapy [41]. Not only does this provide support for the use of progestin-implanted IUDs in the treatment of early hyperplasia, but also suggests the need for more evidence examining the difference in benefits between combined oral contraceptive pills and IUDs and the potential to inform and direct practitioners therapy choices in high-risk populations.

Hormonal Factors

Unopposed Estrogen Therapy

Unopposed estrogen therapy can include estrogens that have varying intensities of effect on end organs. These estrogens can include conjugated equine estrogen (CEE), ethinyl estradiol (EE), micronized 17B-estradiol (E2), along with others. Grady et al. conducted a systematic review of case control and cohort studies in population and hospital based populations and rural and urban populations. She showed that unopposed estrogen users had a relative risk of developing endometrial cancer of 2.3 (95% CI 2.1-2.5) compared to non-users [42]. This risk increased to 9.5 (95%CI 7.4-12.3) in women exposed to unopposed estrogen for 10 or more years. This risk was also dose related (0.3mg CEE RR 3.9 95%CI 1.6-9.5 vs ≥1.25mg CEE RR 5.8 95%CI 4.5-7.5). The risk remained for at least 5 years after use was discontinued. The risk of endometrial cancer death was also increased (RR 2.7, 95%CI 0.9-8.0).

In 2009, Furness reported in the Cochrane Database, a systematic review of randomized studies with unopposed estrogen therapy in postmentopausal women. The outcome of interest was the occurrence of endometrial hyperplasia and/or cancer. They showed that unopposed estrogen was associated with increased risk of endometrial hyperplasia and cancer at all doses and durations of therapy between 1-3 years [43].

Tamoxifen

Tamoxifen is a selective estrogen receptor modulator (SERM) with antiestrogenic properties on breast tissue but estrogenic effects on bone, cardiovascular tissue and the uterus. The National Surgical Adjuvant Breast and Bowel Project (NSABP) B-14 showed that when women with node-negative estrogen receptor positive invasive breast cancer were randomly assigned to placebo (n=1623) versus tamoxifen (20mg/day) (n=1220), the average annual hazard rate for endometrial cancer increased from 0.2/1000 in the placebo group to 1.6/1000 in the tamoxifen group [44]. The relative risk of getting endometrial cancer on tamoxifen was 7.5. They pointed out that this risk of endometrial cancer must be taken into consideration in the context of benefit of tamoxifen against breast cancer relapse i.e., 227.8/1000 in the placebo group to 123.5/1000 in the tamoxifen group. The United States Preventive Services Task Force conducted a systematic review of seven fair to good quality studies comparing tamoxifen, raloxifene and placebo use in women with breast cancer [45]. The risk of tamoxifen associated uterine cancer was 2.13 (95%CI 1.36-3.32) compared to placebo. Raloxifene posed no endometrial cancer risk when compared to placebo and was protective on the uterus when compared to tamoxifen. Breast cancer management has evolved and third generation aromatase inhibitors (anastrozole, letrozole, exemestane) are replacing tamoxifen in about half of the women with breast cancer.

These agents have a lower rate of bleeding and endometrial cancer; however, they cannot be used in premenopausal women [46, 47].

Lifestyle Factors

Obesity

Obesity is one of the most well recognized risk factors for endometrial cancer. It is estimated that obesity is associated with a 2-3 times increased risk of endometrial cancer and this appears to increase with increasing BMI. Crosbie et al. performed a meta-analysis of 24 studies from North America, Europe, Australia, Japan and Korea examining BMI and the risk of endometrial cancer. The study found a relative risk (RR) of 1.6 (95% CI 1.52 - 1.68) for every 5kg/m² increase in BMI. For a BMI of 27 the RR of endometrial cancer was 1.22 (95% CI 1.19 – 1.24) while an individual with a BMI of 42 had almost a 10 times increased risk of endometrial cancer with a RR 9.11 (95% CI 7.26 – 11.51) [48]. Many other studies have replicated these results and have also shown that the association between obesity and endometrial cancer appears to be the greatest when compared to other cancers also thought to be linked to obesity. [48, 49] Renehan et al. performed a systematic review and meta-analysis of 221 data-sets (141 articles) from 1996-2007 and again found a RR of 1.59 (95% CI 1.50 – 1.68). When compared to 20 other major cancers, including gallbladder, esophageal, renal, colon and ovarian, endometrial cancer had the greatest association with BMI [50].

There is debate in the literature over whether childhood and adolescence obesity is a greater risk factor for endometrial cancer versus obesity later in life. While this association appears to hold true for ovarian cancer [51, 52] studies do not show the same for endometrial cancer. Adult weight gain has been shown to have a greater association with endometrial cancer risk than adolescent obesity and studies have also suggested that central obesity may also be an important predictor of risk. More evidence is still required in both areas to determine the degree of these associations [53-56].

There are many different mechanisms by which obesity is thought to increase the risk of endometrial cancer. The most central theory is that obese patients have increased estrogen levels due to conversion of circulating androgens to estrogen by increased aromatase activity in peripheral adipocytes. Obesity is also known to predispose to increased insulin resistance as well as elevated plasma insulin and glucose.

Insulin acts as a growth hormone and may stimulate both ovarian and adrenal androgen synthesis. Insulin may also impact the amount of bioactive IGF-1 which is thought to be related to proliferation of cells and may play a role in the development of hyperplasia [57, 58].

Newer studies have also looked at additional hormones and molecules which may play a role in the association between obesity and endometrial cancer. Both adiponectin and leptin have been shown to be associated with hyperinsulinemia and insulin resistance. Adiponectin is believed to be inversely associated with endometrial cancer while levels of leptin have been shown to be elevated in patients with hyperplasia and endometrial cancer. These hormones may play a role in newer technologies for early detection and management of patients with predisposition to hyperplasia and cancer [59, 57].

Physical Activity

The role of physical activity as a risk factor for endometrial cancer has been debated in the literature. Cust et al. published a literature review in 2007 which examined 18 studies from 11 countries related to activity level and risk for endometrial cancer. Fourteen of the 18 studies showed a protective effect of physical activity with an average relative risk reduction of 30%. Of these a dose response relationship was shown in seven studies. While a positive association has been shown, many of the studies do not adjust for confounding risk factors, particularly obesity and diabetes, two factors thought likely to play a role in the link between physical activity and cancer risk [60]. In 2008, Patel published a prospective cohort study examining 42,672 postmenopausal women with 466 incident cases of endometrial cancer from 1992-2003. Results showed that daily recreational activity resulted in a 30% lower risk of endometrial cancer (RR 0.70 95% CI 0.53-0.93). This was based on comparing one hour of moderate paced walking daily to a sedentary lifestyle. When adjusted for BMI findings were attenuated to a RR of 0.80 (95% CI 0.60

– 1.05) [61]. Furthermore, Friberg in 2006 showed that leisure time inactivity (watching TV or >5 hrs daily sitting) was associated with an increased risk of endometrial cancer with a RR 1.66 (95% CI 1.05-2.61). These findings were also independent of BMI [62].

The biologic mechanisms by which physical activity is thought to reduce the risk of endometrial cancer include the impact on obesity, insulin mediated pathways, immune function and inflammatory pathways. Physical activity has been shown to be associated with improved insulin sensitivity, lower fasting insulin levels and increased SHBG [60, 63, 64,]. Additionally, studies have shown that physical activity influences the circulating levels of anti-inflammatory cytokines [65, 66]. There is increasing evidence that inflammation plays a role in the etiology of endometrial changes. This is believed to occur both by increasing estrogen production as well as altering activation of inflammatory enzymes cyclooxygenase (COX-2) and prostaglandin-E2 in the endometrial tissue [67, 68]. Ultimately, more evidence is still required to determine if and how all of these factors are related in impacting endometrial cancer risk and the optimal types, characteristics and timing of physical activity required to attenuate these risks [60].

Diet

Multiple studies have examined the association between dietary intake and risks of endometrial cancer. Observations have been made linking dietary fat with an increased risk of cancer, while diets high in fruits, vegetables and grains have been thought to lower the risk. Given the association between diabetes, insulin resistance and endometrial cancer, there have also been investigations to determine if diets with a high glycemic load increase the risk of endometrial cancer.

Bravi et al. performed a case-control study of 454 endometrial cancer cases compared to 908 controls in Italy between 1992-2006. Results showed a significant increase in the risk of endometrial cancer for diets high in red meat (OR 2.07;95% CI 1.29-1.33). A reduction in risk was seen for diets high in vegetables and cereals with OR 0.83 (95% CI 0.72-0.95) and 0.91 (95%CI 0.83-0.98) respectively [69]. In a study performed by Cui, high total fat intake was associated with a borderline significant decrease in relative risk (RR 0.78; 95% CI 0.60-0.99, P=0.18), while cereal had a modestly positive association (RR 1.38; 95% CI 1.07-1.79, P=0.05) [70].

Other studies have similarly shown mixed results. A Canadian case-cohort study of 39,614 women published in 2011 showed no significant increase in the risk of endometrial cancer associated with consumption of red meat, while a Danish cohort study of 29,875 women, ages 50-64, between 1993-1997 showed no association between grain, dietary fiber and endometrial cancer. [71-75]. One of the largest studies to date comes from the Women's Health Initiative Dietary Modification Randomized Control Trial in the United States.

This study randomly assigned 48, 835 postmenopausal women to a diet modification intervention versus a usual diet comparison group.

The intervention group had the goal of reducing total fat intake to 20% and increasing consumption of vegetables, fruits and grains. Overall, the risk of endometrial cancer between the two groups did not differ [76].

In terms of high carbohydrate diets, several groups have looked at the association between high glycemic index and cancer risks.

Choi et al. published a meta-analysis of 36 prospective cohort studies examining glycemic index (GI) and glycemic load (GL) in relation to risk of diabetes-related cancers. They defined glycemic index as a unit of measurement used to rank carbohydrate-containing foods (scores ranging from 0 to 100) based on the postprandial blood glucose response compared with an equivalent amount of carbohydrate from a reference food (either glucose or white bread). Glycemic load (GL), on the other hand, is the product of the GI and the grams of carbohydrate content in a serving of a food. In the study there was no significant association with endometrial cancer for the highest versus the lowest GI intake (RR 1.00; 95% CI 0.87 – 1.14). However, the highest category of GL intake was significantly associated with a 21% greater risk of developing endometrial cancer compared with the lowest category of intake (95% CI 1.07-1.37) [77]. A case-control study and meta-analysis of 6 cohort and 2 case-control studies involving 5,569 cases performed by Nagle et al. in Australia reveals similar results. They suggest that the finding of increased risk associated with high glycemic load may signify that the risk is a reflection of both quantity of carbohydrate intake and carbohydrate quality [78].

More research on the impact of diet on endometrial cancer, particularly that of carbohydrates, is needed to determine the extent of the association and the potential to impact changes through lifestyle modification and prevention programs.

Alcohol Consumption

The evidence regarding alcohol consumption and endometrial cancer is inconsistent. Older studies indicated that alcohol may increase the risk of endometrial cancer by increasing circulating estrogen levels [79, 80]. The EPIC (European Prospective Investigation into Cancer and Nutrition) study observed a statistically significant increase in blood oestrone levels among women drinking approximately two drinks per day [81] However, more recent studies have either refuted this hypothesis or considered a dose-dependent relationship. Friberg published a meta-analysis of 7 cohort studies including 1 511 661 participants and 6086 endometrial cancer cases in 2010.

Data showed that compared to non-drinkers, women drinking between half a drink to one drink of alcohol per day had a lower risk of endometrial cancer, while those consuming greater than two drinks per day had up to a 25% increased risk of disease. [82]. These results however did not hold up statistical significance. Furthermore, in 2013, Fedirko reevaluated the data from the EPIC study and looked particularly at rates of endometrial cancer comparing non-drinkers, former drinkers and current drinkers. They found no statistically significant association between alcohol consumption and the risk of endometrial cancer [83].

Cigarette Smoking

The association between cigarette smoking and endometrial cancer is well documented in the literature. Many studies have illustrated a protective effect showing a decrease in risk between 20-50% [84]. One of the largest studies examining smoking and endometrial cancer risk is the Nurse's Health Study in the United States.

The study was a prospective cohort study of 121,700 registered nurses between the ages of 30-55 living in 11 states in the United States. They found that compared to never smokers, current smokers had a RR of endometrial cancer of 0.63 (95% CI 0.50-0.79).

Comparatively, past smokers had a RR of 0.73 (95% CI 0.62 – 0.87). The risk was also found to be lower in those who smoked 35 or more cigarettes per day and among those who smoked for 40 or more years. When adjusting for BMI the relative risk for current smokers was attenuated to a RR of 0.72 (95% 0.57-0.90), however the risk did not change for past smokers [85]. In 2001, Newcomer performed a case control study of Wisconsin women including 740 endometrial cancer cases and 2372 controls. Results showed a RR of 0.8 (95% CI 0.60-1.0) for current smokers compared to those who have never smoked.

The results revealed that smoking also moderates other risk factors for endometrial cancer including obesity, use of post-menopausal hormone and diabetes. There was no effect seen on the association with parity. In this study they did not identify an association with duration, amount smoked, recency or age of starting smoking [84].

The above results indicate that smoking may decrease endometrial cancer risk by also causing a decrease in weight; however the fact that the relative risk remains decreased even after accounting for BMI signifies that there are other biologic mechanisms which may explain this association.

Studies have shown that smoking increases circulating androgens which mitigates the proliferative effects of estrogen. It has also been shown that smoking has toxic effects on the ovaries causing oocyte destruction, decreased levels of estrogen and early menopause. It is most likely a combination of all the above that accounts for the inverse relationship noted in the literature [85].

Medical Factors

Systemic Lupus Erythematous

SLE is one of the most common systemic autoimmune diseases. It often affects people when they are young or middle aged. There is a female preponderance of disease with the ratio of 9 females: 1 male [86]. With the immune role in SLE and autoimmune disease in general (AI) there is an interest in these diseases and their relationship with cancer.

In 2011, Bernatsky et al. conducted a meta-analysis including 5 studies which represented 47,325 male and female SLE patients for 282,553 patient years. There were 66 endometrial cancers for an SIR 0.71 (95% CI 0.55-0.91) [86-88]. One of the hypotheses put forward was that women with SLE have earlier menopause as compared to those without SLE and so this may be responsible for the lower risk of endometrial cancer in this population. In 2012, Hemminki et al. did a population based study in Sweden. They included 4,777,665 person years of which 943 women with AI disorders also developed endometrial cancer. The SIR was significantly decreased at 0.85 [88]. The hypothesis put forward as to why AI disorders are protective against EC include that immunosuppressive therapy may interfere with gonadal steroid synthesis or possibly, that anti-inflammatory medications (ASA, NSAID) may be protective against cancer. The only AI disorder in which the SIR for EC was increased was Hemolytic anemia (SIR 4.11). A hypothesis for this is not clear.

More recently, Bernastky et al. 2013 undertook a multisite international cohort study with 16,409 SLE patients who all met the American College of Rheumatology (ACR) criteria for inclusion [89]. The patients represented US, Canada, Europe and Asia. Their SLE diagnosis was made from 1958-2009. Of the 644 cancers, 12 were endometrial cancers for an SIR 0.44 (95% CI 0.23-0.77). Clearly SLE appears to be protective. The only additional hypothesis put forward in this work involved some genetic predisposition for SLE is protective against EC.

Polycystic Ovarian Syndrome

PCOS is an endocrine disorder of women in the reproductive years. It affects 5-8% of premenopausal women [90]. The first description of polycystic ovary syndrome was made by Stein and Leventhal in 1935 [91]. The association between PCOS and endometrial cancer was first suggested in 1949 by Speert et al. who noted an increased incidence of cystic ovaries in young women with EC [92]. There have been two meta-analyses addressing the relationship between PCOS and EC. Chittenden et al. included four case control studies involving 4056 women (29/56 PCOS patients and 638/4000 control patients developed EC) [93]. They showed that an OR of 2.70 (95% CI 1-7.39) for EC occurring in women with PCOS compared to controls. The EC in the general population was 17 per 100,000 women compared to the rate of 46 per 100,000 in women with PCOS. A second meta-analysis added one study to those in the above meta-analysis [94]. They showed an OR 2.89 (95%CI 1.52-5.48) and a 9% lifetime risk of EC in women with PCOS compared to 3% in women from the general population.

Although there are many published case control and cohort studies, one of the common problems these authors found in conducting their meta-analysis was that many studies lacked clear criteria for diagnosing PCOS.

Many studies looked at anovulation and not PCOS, or they included women who made a personal report of the condition rather than confirming the diagnosis biochemically or using standard diagnosis.

The mortality rate for women with PCOS and EC appears lower than that of the general population. For example, Pierpoint followed 786 women diagnosed as PSOC in the UK hospital records from 1930-1979. The mortality rate in those who developed EC was not increased. This was suggested to be related to the fact EC in PCOS women are usually well differentiated [95, 96].

There is a complex relationship between PCOS and EC as they share similar risk factors i.e., obesity, type 2 diabetes, hypertension, anovulation, and nulliparity. For example, women with PCOS have a 5-10 fold increased risk of type 2 diabetes while women with EC have a 3 fold increased risk. In fact, the strength of the association between PCOS and EC actually drops when confounding like body mass index is taken into account [97]. An Australian study showed the association of PCOS and EC compared to women without PCOS was 4.0 (95% CI 1.7-9.3). When adjusted for BMI the OR dropped to 2.2 (95%CI 0.9-5.7). Thus, whether the risk factor is PCOS or rather a confounder is not yet clear. The association between PCOS and EC could be explained by several endocrine, metabolic and anthropomorphic features of PCOS which are recognized risk factors for EC [98]. For example, oligo or amenorrhea can result in prolonged estrogen stimulation of endometrium which when unopposed by progesterone can lead to hyperplasia and EC.

Hypersecretion of LH is seen in 65% of women with PCOS while in endometrial hyperplasia and cancer there is an overexpression of LH and FSH receptors in endometrium. Women with PCOS are more likely to have insulin resistance even after adjusting for BMI. Insulin upregulates aromatase activity in endometrial epithelial and stromal cell cultures.

Thus estrogen from circulating androgens may be enhanced. IGF-1 which is enhanced in PCOS also accelerates growth of EC cells. Androgens are stimulatory to endometrial cells. Genes involved in carcinogenesis appeared to be switched on at an earlier level in histologically normal women who did not cycle regularly i.e., bcl-2, bax., CYR61, Ki67, cFos.

Diabetes

Several studies have shown a higher risk of endometrial cancer among diabetic patients. What remains less clear is whether this is an independent association or secondary to weight. A meta-analysis by Zhang et al. in 2012 analyzed 21 cohort studies involving 12,195 incident cases and 575 deaths caused by endometrial cancer from 8 different countries. Results showed diabetes was associated with an increased incidence of endometrial cancer. (RR 1.81; 95% CI 1.38-2.37.) However, few of the studies included controlled for BMI directly. In this study there was no positive association between diabetes and endometrial cancer mortality, which has been replicated in a number of other studies [99, 100]. In 2012, the National Institutes of Health-American Association of Retired Persons (NIH-AARP) diet and health study was published. This prospective cohort study followed 199,591 women from 6 states in the United States. They completed a questionnaire in 1995-1996 and then were followed up through 2006. The study found that overweight and obese participants with diabetes had a higher risk of endometrial cancer than overweight and obese patients without diabetes.

For patients with a BMI of 30-35 the HR for endometrial cancer incidence among patients without diabetes was 2.09 (95% CI 1.71-2.55) compared to a HR of 2.62 (95% CI 1.88-3.65) for those patients with diabetes [101].

This positive association has been reinforced by studies of metformin which suggest that this oral hypoglycemic medication may decrease rates of endometrial cancer.

Molecular studies have shown metformin to induce apoptosis and prevent cellular proliferation in type I endometrial cancer cell lines [102]. A recent study in Israel also demonstrated that metformin interacts with the IGF pathway and induced apoptosis in uterine serous carcinoma cell lines [58].

Conclusion

The global profile of endometrial cancer shows higher incidence rates in more developed countries, and advanced age (after menopause). Other work has shown increased incidence of disease in women who carry certain genetic mutations like Lynch syndrome (MSH2, MLH1, MSH6, PMS2), nulliparity, infertility, exposure to certain homones (unopposed estrogen therapy, tamoxifen), obesity, diabetes and polycystic ovary syndrome. Factors that appear to be protective include oral contraception use, IUDs and medicated IUDs, physical activity, smoking, and immune conditions like systemic lupus erythe-matous.

Epidemiologic studies help researchers focus their questions on biologic mechanisms for disease which could be exploited in either treatment (progesterone use for women with grade 1 metastatic endometrial cancer) or prevention (progesterone use in women with endometrial hyperplasia). The role of diet, exercise and agents like metformin in preventing endometrial cancer or survivorship after being diagnosed with disease continues to require further evaluation.

References

Introduction

[1] Prat, J., Gallardo, A., Cuatrecasas, M., et al. Endometrial carcinoma: Pathology and genetics. *Pathology* 2007;39:1-7.

[2] Setiawan, V. W., Yang, H. P., Pike, M. C., et al. Type I and II endometrial cancers: Have they different risk factors? *J. Clin. Oncol.* 2013; 31(20): 2607-2618.

[3] Brinton, L. A., Felix, A. S., McMeekin, S., et al. Etiologic heterogeneity in endometrial cancer: Evidence from a Gynecologic Oncology Group trial. *Gynecol. Oncol.* 2013;129:277-284.

[4] Yang, H. P., Wentzensen, N., Trabert, B., et al. Endometrial cancer risk factors by 2 main histologic subtypes: The NIH-AARP Diet and Health Study. *Am. J. Epidemiol.* 2013;177(2):142-151.

[5] Parazzini, F., LaVecchia, C., Bocciolone, L., et al. The epidemiology of endometrial cancer. *Gynecol. Oncol.* 1991;41:1-16.

[6] Globocan 2008. *Fact Sheets.* http://globocan.iarc.fr/. June 10, 2013.

[7] Howlader, N., Noone, A. M., Krapcho, M., et al. *SEER Cancer Statistics Review, 1975-2010*, National Cancer Institute. Bethesda, MD, http://seer.cancer.gov/csr/1975_2010/, based on November 2012 SEER data submission, posted to the SEER web site, 2013.

Genetics

[8] Taylor, N., Mutch, D. G. Gynecologic manifestations of hereditary non-polyposis colon cancer. From inherited to sporadic disease. *Oncolgy* (Williston Park) 2006;1:85-94.

[9] Wijnin, J., de Leeuw, W., Vasen, H., et al. Familial endometrial cancer in female carriers of MSH6 germline mutations. *Nat. Genet.* 1999;23: 142-144

[10] Hampel, H., Frankel, W., Panescu, J., et al. Screening for Lynch syndrome (hereditary nonpolyposis colon cancer) among endometrial cancer patients. *Cancer Res.* 2006;15:7810-7817.

[11] Hampel, H., Panescu, J., Lockman, J., et al. (Comment on) Screening for Lynch syndrome (hereditary nonpolypois colon cancer) among endometrial cancer patients. *Cancer Res.* 2007;62:9603.

[12] Karlan, B., Berchuk, A., Mutch, D. The role of genetic testing for cancer susceptibility in gynecologic practice. *Obstet. Gynecol.* 2007;110:155-167.

[13] Dunlop, M. G., Farrington, S. M., Carothers, A. D., et al. Cancer risk associated with germline DNA mismatch repair gene mutations. *Hum. Mol. Genet.* 1997;6:105-110.

[14] Aarnio, M., Sankila, R., Pukkala, E., et al. Cancer risk in mutation carriers of DNA-mismatch-repair genes. *Int. J. Cancer* 1999;81(2):214-218.

[15] Vasen, H. F., Wijnen, J. T., Menko, F. H., et al. Cancer risk in families with hereditary nonpolyposis colorectal cancer diagnosed by mutation analysis. *Gastroenterology* 1996;110(4):1020-1027.

[16] Hendriks, Y. M., Wagner, A., Morreau, H., et al. Cancer risk in hereditary nonpolyposis colorectal cancer due to MSH6 mutations: impact on counselling and surveillance. *Gastroenterology* 2004;127(1):17-25.

[17] Hampel, H., Stephens, J. A., Pukkala, E., et al. Cancer risk in hereditary nonpolyposis colorectal cancer syndrome: later age of onset. *Gastroenterology* 2005;129(2):415-442.

[18] Boilesen, A. E. B., Bisgaard, M. L., Bernstein, I. Risk of gynecologic cancers in Danish hereditary non polyposis colorectal cancer families. *Acta Obstet. Gynecol.* 2008;87:1127-1135.

[19] Schmeler, K. M., Lu, K. H. Gynecologic cancers associated with Lynch Ssyndrome/HNPCC. *Clin. Transl. Oncol.* 2008;10:313-317.

[20] Dove-Edwin, I., Boks, D., Goff, S., et al. The outcome of endometrial carcinoma surveillance by ultrasound scan in women at risk of hereditary nonpolyposis colorectal carcinoma and familial colorectal carcinoma. *Cancer* 2002;94:1708-1712.

[21] Rijcken, F. E., Mourits, M. J., Kleibeuker, J. H., et al. Gynecologic screening in hereditary nonpolyposis colorectal cancer. *Gynecol. Oncol.* 2003;91:73-80.

[22] Reckonen-Sinisalo, L., Butzow, R., Leminen, A., et al. Surveillance for endometrial cancer in hereditary nonpolyposis colorectal cancer syndrome. *Int. J. Cancer* 2007;120;821-824.

[23] Schmeler, K., Lynch, H., Chen, L., et al. Prophylactic surgery to reduce the risk of gynecologic cancers in the Lynch syndrome. *N. Engl. J. Med.* 2006;354:261-269.

[24] Daniels, M., Schmeler, K. W. P., Chen, L., et al. Clinical and pathologic features of ovarian cancer in women with Lynch syndrome mutations.

Proceedings of the 2nd Biennial scientific Meeting of Int Society of GI Hereditary Tumors. (InSiGHT Japan) 2007.

[25] Hornreich, G., Beller, U., Lavie, O., et al. Is uterine serous papillary carcinoma a BRCA1 related disease? Case report and review of the literature. *Gynecol. Oncol.* 1999;75:300-304.

[26] Levine, D., Lin, O., Barakat, R., et al. Risk of endometrial cancer associated with BRCA mutation. *Gynecol. Oncol.* 2001;80:395-398.

[27] Goshen, R., Chu, W., Elit, L., et al. Is uterine papillary serous adeno-carcinoma a manifestation of the hereditary breast-ovarian cancer syndrome? *Gynecol. Oncol.* 2000 Dec.;79(3):477-481.

[28] Beiner, M., Fich, A., Rosen, A., et al. The risk of endometrial cancer in women with BRCA1 and BRCA2 mutations. A prospective study. *Gynecol. Oncol.* 2007;104:7-10.

Reproductive Factors

[29] Albrektsen, G., Heuch, I., Tretli, S., et al. Is the risk of cancer of the corpus uteri reduced by a recent pregnancy? A prospective study of 765, 756 Norwegian women. *Int. J. Cancer* 1995;61(4):485–490.

[30] Bevier, M., Sundquist, J., Hemminki, K. Does the time interval between first and last birth influence the risk of endometrial and ovarian cancer? *Eur. J. Cancer* 2011;47:586-591.

[31] Setiawan, V. W., Pike, M. C., Karageorgi, S., et al. Age at last birth in relation to risk of endometrial cancer: Pooled analysis in the epidemiology of endometrial cancer consortium. *Am. J. Epidemiol.* 2012; 176(4): 269-278.

[32] Dossus, L., Allen, N., Kaaks, R., et al. Reproductive risk factors and endometrial cancer: The European Prospective Investigation into Cancer and Nutrition. *Int. J. Cancer* 2010; 127: 442-451.

[33] Xu, W. H., Xiang, Y. B., Ruaz, Zx., et al. Menstrual and reproductive factors and endometrial cancer risk: results from a population-based case-control study in urban Shanghai. *Int. J. Cancer* 2004; 108: 613-619.

[34] Modan, B., Ron, E., Lerner-Geva, L., et al. Cancer incidence in a cohort of infertile women. *Am. J. Epidemiol.* 1998;147(11):1038–1042.

[35] Althius, M. D., Moghissi, K. S., Westhoff, C. L., et al. Uterine cancer after use of clomiphene citrate to induce ovulation. *Am. J. Epidemiol.* 2005; 161(7): 607-615.

[36] Brinton, L. A., Westhoff, C. L., Scoccia, B., et al. Fertility drugs and endometrial cancer risk: results from an extended follow-up of a large infertility cohort. *Human Reproduction* 2013; 0(0): 1-9.

[37] Maxwell, G. L., Schildkraut, J. M., Calingaert, B., et al. Progestin and estrogen potency of combination oral contraceptives and endometrial cancer risk. *Gynecol. Oncol.* 2006;103(2):535–540.

[38] Weiderpass, E., Adami, H. O., Baron, J. A., et al. Use of oral contraceptives and endometrial cancer risk (Sweden). *Cancer Causes Control* 1999;10(4):277–284.

[39] Cramer, D. W. The epidemiology of endometrial and ovarian cancer. *Hematol. Oncol. Clin. N. Am.* 2012: 26;1-12.

[40] Beining, R. M., Dennis, L. K., Smith, E. M., et al. Meta-analysis of intrauterine device use and risk of endometrial cancer. *Ann. Epidemiol.* 2008; 18:492-499.

[41] Orbo, A., Rise, C. E., Mutter, G. L. Regression of latent endometrial precancers by progestin infiltrated intrauterine device. *Cancer Res.* 2006;66:5613-5617.

Hormonal Factors

[42] Grady, D., Gebretsadik, T., Ernster, V., et al. Hormone replacement therapy and endometrial cancer risk: a meta-analysis. *Obstet. Gynecol.* 1995;85:304-313.

[43] Furness, S., Roberts, H., Marjoribanks, J., et al. Hormone therapy in postmenopausal women and risk of endometrial hyperplasia. *Cochrane Database Syst. Rev.* 2009;15(2):CD000402.

[44] Fisher, B., Costantino, J. P., Redmond, K. C., et al. Endometrial cancer in tamoxifen-treated breast cancer patients: findings from the National Surgical Adjuvant Breast and Bowel Project (NSABP) B-14. *J. Natl. Cancer Inst.* 1994;86:527-537.

[45] Nelson, H. D., Smith, M. E. B., Griffin, J. C., et al. Use of medications to reduce risk for primary breast cancer: a systematic review for the US Preventive services task force. *Ann. Int. Med.* 2013;158:604-614.

[46] Breast International Group 1-98 Collaborative Group. A comparison of letrozole and tamoxifen in postmenopausal women with early breast cancer. *N. Engl. J. Med.* 2005;35:2747-2757.

[47] Kaufmann, M., Jonat, W., Hilfrich, J., et al. Improved overall survival in postmenopausal women with early breast cancer after anastozole

initiated after 2 years of treatment with tamoxifen compared with continued tamoxifen: the ARNO 95 study. *J. Clin. Oncol.* 2007;24:2664-2670.

Lifestyle Factors

[48] Crosbie, E. J., Zwahlen, M., Kitchener, H. C., et al. Body mass index, hormone replacement therapy and endometrial cancer risk: a meta-analysis. *Cancer Epidemiol. Biomarkers Prev.* 2010;19 (12):3119-3130.
[49] Renehan, A., Tyson, M., Egger, M., Heller, R. F., et al. Body mass index and incidence of cancer: a systematic review and meta-analysis of prospective observational studies. *Lancet* 2008; 371: 569-78.
[50] Calle, E. E., Rodriguez, C., Walker-Thurmond, K., et al. Overweight, obesity and mortality from cancer in a prospectively studied cohort of US adults. *N. Engl. J. Med.* 2003; 348:1625.
[51] Fairfield, K. M., Willett, W. C., Rosner, B. A., et al. Obesity, weight gain, and ovarian cancer. *Obstet. Gynecol.* 2002;100:288.
[52] Engeland, A., Treti, S., Bjorge, T. Height, body mass index and ovarian cancer: a follow-up of 1.1 million Norwegian women. *J. Natl. Cancer Inst.* 2003; 95:1244.
[53] Friedenreich, C., Cust, A., Lahmann, P. H., et al. Anthropometric factors and risk of endometrial cancer: the European prospective investigation into cancer and nutrition. *Cancer Causes Control* 2007;18:399-413.
[54] Schmandt, R. E., Iglesias, D. A., Co, N. N., et al. Understanding obesity and endometrial cancer risk: opportunities for prevention. *Am. J. Obstet. Gynecol.* 2011;205:518-525.
[55] Yang, T. Y., Cairns, B. J., Allen, N., et al. Postmenopausal endometrial cancer risk and body size in early life and middle age: prospective cohort study. *Br. J. Cancer* 2012;107(1):169-175.
[56] Chang, S. C., Lacey, J. V. Jr. Lifetime weight history and endometrial cancer risk by type of menopausal hormone use in the NIH-AARP diet and health study. *Cancer Epidemiol. Biomarkers Prev.* 2007;16: 723-730.
[57] Nickles Fader, A., Nieves Arriba, L., Fraser, H. E., et al. Endometrial cancer and obesity: Epidemiology, biomarkers, prevention and survivorship. *Gynecol. Oncol.* 2009; 114: 121-127.
[58] Sarfstein, R., Friedman, Y., Attias-Geva, Z., et al. Metformin down-regulates the insulin/IGF-I signaling pathway and inhibits different

uterine serous carcinoma (USC) cells proliferation and migration in p53-dependend or – independent manners. *PLoS One* 2013; 8(4):e61537.
[59] Yurkovetsky, Z., Ta'asan, S., Skates, S., et al. Development of multi-marker panel for early detection of endometrial cancer. High diagnostic power of prolactin. *Gynecol. Oncol.* 2007; 107: 58-65.
[60] Cust, A. E., Armstrong, B. K., Friedenreich, C. M., et al. Physical activity and endometrial cancer risk: a review of the current evidence, biologic mechanisms and the quality of physical activity assessment methods. *Cancer Causes Control* 2007;18(3):243–258.
[61] Patel, A. V., Feigelson, H. S., Talbot, J. T., et al. The role of body weight in the relationship between physical activity and endometrial cancer: Results from a large cohort of US women. *Int. J. Cancer* 2008; 123: 1877-1882.
[62] Friberg, E., Mantzoros, C. S., Wolk, A. Physical activity and risk of endometrial cancer: a population-based prospective cohort study. *Cancer Epidemiol. Biomarkers Prev.* 2006;15(11):2136–2140.
[63] Mayer-Davis, E. J., D'Agostino, R. Jr, Karter, A. J., et al. Intensity and amount of physical activity in relation to insulin sensitivity: the Insulin Resistance Atherosclerosis Study. *JAMA* 1998; 279:669–674.
[64] Borghouts, L. B., Keizer, H. A. Exercise and insulin sensitivity: a review. *Int. J. Sports Med.* 2000; 21:1–12.
[65] Moldoveanu, A. I., Shephard, R. J., Shek, P. N. The cytokine response to physical activity and training. *Sports Med.* 2001; 31:115–144.
[66] Pischon, T., Hankinson, S. E., Hotamisligil, G. S., et al. Leisure-time physical activity and reduced plasma levels of obesity-related inflammatory markers. *Obes. Res.* 2003; 11:1055–1064.
[67] Purohit, A., Newman, S. P., Reed, M. J., The role of cytokines in regulating estrogen synthesis: implications for the etiology of breast cancer. *Breast Cancer Res.* 2002; 4:65–69.
[68] Modugno, F., Ness, R. B., Chen, C., et al. Inflammation and endometrial cancer: a hypothesis. *Cancer Epidemiol. Biomarkers Prev.* 2005;14: 2840–2847.
[69] Bravi, F., Scotti, L., Bosetti, C., et al. Food groups and endometrial cancer risk: a case-control study from Italy. *Am. J. Obstet. Gynecol.* 2009; 200(3): 293.e1-7.
[70] Cui, X., Rosner, B., Willett, W. C., et al. Dietary fat, fiber, and carbohydrate intake in relation to risk of endometrial cancer. *Cancer Epidemiol. Biomarkers Prev.* 2011;20:978-989.

[71] Jain, M. G., Rohan, T. E., Howe, G. R., et al. A cohort study of nutriational factors and endometrial cancer. *Eur. J. Epidemiol.* 2000; 16: 899-905.
[72] Van, L. L., Kirsh, V. A., Kreiger, N., et al. Endometrial cancer and meat consumption: a case-cohort study. *Eur. J. Cancer Prev.* 2011;20:334-339.
[73] Barbone, F., Austin, H., Partridge, E. E. Diet and endometrial cancer: a case-control study. *Am. J. Epidemiol.* 1993;137:393-403.
[74] Goodman, M. T., Hankin, J. H., Wilkens, L. R., et al. Diet, body size, physical activity, and the risk of endometrial cancer. *Cancer Res.* 1997; 57: 5077-5085.
[75] Aarestrup, J., Kryo, C., Christensen, J., et al. Whole grain, dietary fiber and incidence of endometrial cancer in a Danish cohort study. *Nutr. Cancer* 2012; 64(8): 1160-1168.
[76] Prentice, R. L., Thomson, C. A., Caan, B., et al. Low-fat dietary pattern and cancer incidence in the Women's Health Initiative Dietary Modification Randomized Controlled Trial. *J. Natl. Cancer Inst.* 2007; 99:1534-1543.
[77] Choi, Y., Givannucci, E., Lee, Je. Glycemic index and glycemic load in relation to risk of diabetes related cancers: a meta-analysis. *Br. J. Nutr.* 2012; 108:1934-1947.
[78] Nagel, C. M., Olsen, C. M., Ibiebele, T. I., et al. Glycemic index, glycemic load and endometrial cancer risk: results from the Australian National Endometrial Cancer study and an updated systematic review and meta-analysis. *Eur. J. Nutr.* 2013;52(5):705-715.
[79] Gavaler, J. S., Van Thiel, D. H. The association between moderate alcoholic beverage consumption and serum estradiol and testosterone levels in normal postmenopausal women: relationship to the literature. *Alcohol Clin. Exp. Res.* 1992;16:87 – 92.
[80] Hankinson, S. E., Willett, W. C., Manson, J. E., Hunter, D. J., Colditz, G. A., Stampfer, M. J., Longcope, C., Speizer, F. E. Alcohol, height, and adiposity in relation to estrogen and prolactin levels in postmenopausal women. *J. Natl. Cancer Inst.* 1995;87:1297 – 1302.
[81] Rinaldi, S., Peeters, P. H., Dossus, L., et al. Relationship of alcohol intake and sex steroid concentrations in blood in pre- and postmenpausal women: the European Prospective Investigation into Cancer and Nutrition. *Cancer Causes Control* 2006; 17: 1033 – 1043.

[82] Friberg, E., Orsini, N., Mantxoros, C. S., et al. Alcohol intake and endometrial cancer risk: a meta-analysis of prospective studies. *Br. J. Cancer* 2010;103:127-131.

[83] Fedirko, V., Jenab, M., Rinaldi, S., et al. Alcohol drinking and endometrial cancer risk in the European Prospective Investigation into Cancer and Nutrition (EPIC) Study. *Ann. Epidemiol.* 2013; 23: 93-98.

[84] Newcomer, L. M., Newcomb, P. A., Trentham-Dietz, et al. Hormonal risk factors for endometrial cancer: Modifications by cigarette smoking. *Cancer Causes and Control* 2001:12:829-835.

[85] Viswanathan, A. N., Feskanich, D., De Vivo, et al. Smoking and the risk of endometrial cancer: results from the Nurses' Health Study. *Int. J. Cancer* 2005; 114: 996-1001.

Medical Factors

[86] Bernatsky, S., Ramsey-Goldman, R., Foulkes, W., et al. Breast, ovarian and endometrial malignancies in systemic lupus erythematosus: a meta-analysis. *Br. J. Cancer* 2011;104:1478-1481.

[87] Bernatsky, S., Kale, M., Ramsey-Goldman, R., Gordon, C., et al. Systemic lupus and malignancies. *Rhematology* 2012;24(2):177-181.

[88] Hemminki, K., Liu, X., Ji, J., et al. Effect of autoimmune diseases on risk and survival in female cancers. *Gynecol. Oncol.* 2012;127:180-185.

[89] Bernatsky, S., Ramsey-Goldman, R., Labrecque, J., et al. Cancer risk in systemic lupus: An updated international multi-centre cohort study. *J. Autoimmunity.* 2013;42:130-135.

[90] Fanta, M. Is polycystic ovary sundrome a state of relative extrogen excess, a real risk factor for estrogen-dependant malignancies? *Gynecol. Endomcrin.* 2013;29(2):145-147.

[91] Stein, I. F., Leventhal, M. L. Amenorrhea associated with bilateral poly-cystic ovaries. *Am. J. Obstet. Gynecol.* 1935;25:181-191.

[92] Speert, H. Carcinoma of the endometrium in young women. *Surg. Gynecol. Obstet.* 1949;88:332-336.

[93] Chittenden, B. C., Fullerton, G., Maheshwari, A., et al. Polycystic ovary sundreom and the risk of gynaecological cancer: a systematic review. *Reprod. Biomed. Online* 2009;19:398-405.

[94] Haoula, Z., Salman, M., Atiomo, W. Evaluating the association between endometrial cancer and polycystic ovarian syndrome. *Hum. Reprod.* 2012;27:1327-1331.

[95] Pierdpoint, T., McKeigue, P. M., Isaacs, A. J., et al. Mortality of women with polycystic ovary syndrome at long-term follow-up. *J. Clin. Epidemiol.* 1998;51:581-586.

[96] Jafari, K., Javaheri, G., Ruiz, G., Endometrial adenocarcinoma and the Stein-Leventhal syndrome. *Obstet. Gyneol.* 1978;51:97-100.

[97] Fearnley, E. J., Marquart, L., Spurdle, A. B., et al. The Ausralian OvarianCancer Study Group and The Australian National Endometrial Cancer Study Group. Polycystic ovary syndrome increases the risk of endometrial cancer in women aged less than 50 years: an Australian case-control study. *Cancer Causes Control* 2010;21:2303-2308.

[98] Navaratnarajah, R., Pillay, O. C., Hardiman, P. Polycystic Ovary Sundrome and endometrial cancer. *Semin. Reprod. Med.* 2008;26(1):62-71.

[99] Zhang, Z. H., Su, P. Y., Hao, J. H., et al. The role of preexisting diabetes mellitus on incidence and mortality of endometrial cancer. A meta-analysis of prospective cohort studies. *Int. J. Gynecol. Cancer* 2013; 23 (2): 294-303.

[100] Chia, V. M., Newcomb, P. A., Trentham-Dietz, A., et al. Obesity, diabetes and other factors in relation to survival after endometrial cancer diagnosis. *Int. J. Gynecol. Cancer* 2007;17:441-446.

[101] Lai, G. Y., Park, Y., Hartge, P., et al. The Association between self-reported diabetes and cancer incidence in the NIH-AARP Diet and Health Study. *J. Clin. Endocrinol. Metab.* 2013;98(3): F497-F502.

[102] Cantrell, L. A., Zhou, C., Mendivil, A., et al. Metformin is a potent inhibitor of endometrial cancer cell proliferation-implications for a novel treatment strategy. *Gynecol. Oncol.* 2010;116: 92–98.

In: Endometrial Cancer
Editors: I. Diaz-Padilla, J. Garcia-Donas
ISBN: 978-1-63321-323-4

Chapter II

Inherited Predisposition to Endometrial Cancer

***Ignacio Romero Noguera*[1] *and Zaida García-Casado*[2]**

[1]Clinical Area Gynecologic Oncology, Instituto Valenciano de Oncologia, Valencia, Spain

[2]Laboratory of Molecular Biology, Instituto Valenciano de Oncologia, Valencia, Spain

"The *family* tree *has become the most important genetic test* of all. The more you know the more tools you have to practice preventive medicine."

Donna Russo, coordinator of the cancer genetics program at New York-Presbyterian Hospital.

Introduction

Identifying inherited predisposition to endometrial cancer (EC) syndromes can help cancer patients prevent secondary malignancies and identify family members who may be at risk in order to initiate a screening protocol. The first step must include a comprehensive family history assessment to identify the family syndrome and performing a molecular testing according to the findings since several inherited predisposition syndromes have been identified.

Lynch syndrome is the most common hereditary cause of colorectal and endometrial cancer in women. It accounts for 2% to 4% of all colorectal cancers and 2% to 5% of endometrial cancers in women [1]. Cowden Syndrome (CS) is also associated to EC, female and male breast cancer and thyroid cancer with benign features including patognomic criteria such as Lhermitte-Duclos disease, dysplastic gangliocytoma of the cerebellum and cutaneous manifestations including facial trichilemmoma, acral keratosis, papillomatous papules and mucosal lesions with well-established criteria for identification [2]. Germline mutations in *PTEN* account for 80% and recently a CS and CS-like without *PTEN* mutations enriched in kidney cancer in an overlapping syndrome with familial paraganglioma syndromes were identified with *SDHB* or *SDHD* germline mutations [3]. Uterine leiomyosarcomas as a soft tissue sarcoma can occur in Li Fraumeni (*TP53* germline mutation) syndrome [4].

Uterine serous carcinoma is underrepresented in LS, and there is still controversy over whether it belongs to LS or Hereditary Breast and Ovarian carcinoma. Recent data have found Germline mutations [5] in *BRCA1* (2.0%), *TP53* (1.3%) and CHEK2 (1.3%).

Lynch Syndrome

Definition

LS originally called hereditary nonpolyposis colorectal cancer (HNPCC), is an autosomal dominant cancer predisposition syndrome [6]. LS is now the common accepted designation and should be reserved for cases where there is molecular evidence of a germline Mistmatch Repair Defect (MMR) [7]. When this is not the case we can only suspect it and it has proven to be a source of difficulties in interpreting publications as will be seen later. It is characterized by more frequent and early onset of colorectal, endometrial, ovarian, gastric, ureter and renal pelvis, biliary tract, brain, pancreatic and small bowel cancers as well as sebaceous gland adenomas and keratoachantomas as seen in Muir-Torre syndrome.

Identification Criteria

Several strategies used to identify LS patients will be reviewed. Those include clinical identification criteria, estimation models for predicting mutation carrier probabilities, pathologic identification criteria and molecular screening tools.

Whether a single or combined approach or universal screening is the most appropriate identification technique will be covered in this chapter.

Clinical Identification Criteria

Universal criteria: When working with these criteria we have to bear in mind that they were initially developed to identify colorectal cancer (CRC) patients as it is the most common cancer syndrome but in women EC can appear earlier than CRC [8]. Although Amsterdam I criteria included only CRC, Amsterdam II [9] (table 1) and revised Bethesda [10] (table 2) guidelines include all LS spectrum of cancers.

The Society of Gynecologic Oncology (SGO) has developed criteria [11] (table 3 and 4) to help gynecologic oncologists identify EC as red flag for LS based on young onset, synchronous or metachronous cancers and family history.

Synchronicity: Since ovarian cancer also belongs to LS and synchronous endometrial cancers occurs in 5-10% of cases, the feature selection strategy has been investigated. Soliman [12] reports that 7% met either clinical or molecular criteria for Lynch syndrome and all had family members with LS associated cancers or a personal history of such cancers while in another series [13] 9% had a loss of MLH1, MSH2 or MSH6 tumor staining and all had a family history of cancer. Another study found that clear cell histology in both ovary and endometrium should raise suspicion of LS [14].

Young age: Another approach is selecting EC patients younger than 50 years regardless of their family history. In the two studies [15, 16] that examined this, 8-9% were *MLH1*, *MSH2* or *MSH6* mutation carriers. In the study by Lu they further examined the impact of body mass index (BMI) –a well-established risk factor for EC- and found that mutation carriers had a lower BMI compared with non-carriers. The BMI analysis in carriers and non-carriers in an epidemiologic study suggested an obesity-independent endometrial carcinogenesis for carriers [17]. Another study [18] selected a cut off of less than 40 years yielding 16% loss of MMR proteins in immunohistochemistry (IHC). Hampel [19] found that in 543 EC patients unselected for family history, in the cohort of patients less than 50 years 5% had LS with germline deleterious mutation in MMR genes. Therefore, selecting young EC patients for additional tumor studies is an approach which could help increase detection rate. While the median age of onset of LS-EC is 47 years, according to the type of Germline mutations, it can vary between 49,

46, 51 and 64 in respectively *MLH1*, *MSH2*, *MSH6* and *PMS2* [20]. A younger cut off would leave some patients unidentified if criteria of age is the only approach.

Limitations: although these are well established criteria, in real life setting, a comprehensive family history is not always sought. Knowing that these criteria are not easily recognizable has raised awareness in this area. Some believe that this should prompt more automated, easy to perform screening tests to identify EC associated to LS such as universal IHC screening.

In an Australian [21] study only 26% of EC patients had family history properly annotated in medical records, and only 6% and 14% of cases fulfilling respectively rBC and AII criteria were referred for Genetic Counseling.

They were more likely to be referred if the red flags for LS are commonly identified such as: two first- or second-degree relatives diagnosed with Lynch associated cancers, cancer in a family member diagnosed before age 50, or three first-degree relatives with LS associated cancers.

Moreover, in a well identified cohort of EC patients with complete family records and MMR study, [22] clinical criteria were only able to identify families at risk in 36%, 58%, 71% and 93% with rBC, AmII, SGO 20%-to-25%, and SGO 5%-to-10% criteria.

Estimation Models for Prediction

Free access software models (table 5) for predicting the probability of index cases of carrying a germline mutation based on different variables of personal and family history have been presented.

They were initially developed and have been validated for colorectal cancer (CRC).

These tools help clinicians select patients for further testing for LS.

Table 1. Amsterdam II criteria (AII): Patients must meet all of the following

At least three relatives must have a cancer associated with LS (colorectal, cancer of endometrium, small bowel, ureter, or renal-pelvis):
One must be a first-degree relative of the other two;
At least two successive generations must be affected;
At least one relative with cancer associated with LS should be diagnosed before age 50 years;
FAP should be excluded in the CRC case(s) (if any);
Tumors should be verified whenever possible

Table 2. Revised Bethesda Criteria (rBC): Guidelines for testing Microsatellite Instability

CRC diagnosed in a patient who is younger than 50 years of age.
Presence of synchronous, or metachronous, colorectal or other LS-related tumors regardless of age.
CRC with the MSI-H histology diagnosed in a patient who is younger than 60 years of age.
CRC diagnosed in a patient with one or more first-degree relatives with an LS-related cancer, with one of the cancers being diagnosed under age 50 years.
CRC diagnosed in a patient with two or more first- or second-degree relatives with LS-related cancer regardless of age

MSI-H histology is defined by the presence of tumor infiltrating lymphocytes, Crohn's-like lymphocytic reaction, mucinous/signet-ring differentiation, or medullary growth pattern.

Note: LS-related cancers include colorectal, endometrial, ovarian, gastric, ureter and renal pelvis, biliary tract, brain, pancreatic and small bowel cancers as well as sebaceous gland adenomas and keratoachantomas as seen in Muir-Torre syndrome.

Table 3. Patients with greater than approximately 20-25% chance of having inherited predisposition to endometrial, colorectal, and related cancers and for whom genetic risk assessment is recommended

Women with a personal history of both breast and ovarian cancer
Women with ovarian cancer and a close relative with breast cancer at ≤50 years or ovarian cancer at any age
Women with ovarian cancer at any age who are of Ashkenazi Jewish ancestry
Women with breast cancer at ≤50 years and a close relative with ovarian or male breast cancer at any age
Women of Ashkenazi Jewish ancestry and breast cancer at≤40 years
Women with a 1st or 2nd degree relative with a knownBRCA1 or BRCA2 mutation

$PREMM_{1,2,6}$ model [23] (prediction of mismatch repair gene mutations in *MLH1*, *MSH2*, and *MSH6*) includes variables such as gender, history and ages of CRC and EC, and history of other LS-associated cancers. Family history data included the number of first-and second-degree relatives with a history of CRC, EC, and other LS-associated tumors, as well as the youngest ages of diagnosis of CRC and EC. Predicted genes are MLH1, MSH2 and MSH6. It is based on data supplied on the test submission forms for Myriad Genetics Inc.

Table 4. Patients with greater than approximately 5% to 10% chance of having an inherited predisposition to endometrial, colorectal, and related cancers and for whom genetic risk may be helpful

Women with breast cancer at ≤40 years
Women with bilateral breast cancer (particularly if the first cancer was at ≤50 years)
Women with breast cancer at ≤50 years and a close relative with breast cancer at ≤50 years
Women of Ashkenazi Jewish ancestry with breast cancer at ≤50 years
Women with breast or ovarian cancer at any age and two or more close relatives with breast cancer at any age (particularly if at least 1 breast cancer was at ≤50 years)
Unaffected women with a 1st or 2nd degree relative that meets one of the above criteria

MMR predict model [24] variables include age at diagnosis of CRC, gender, location of tumor (proximal versus distal), synchronous or metachronous tumors, history and youngest age of diagnosis of CRC in first-degree relatives, and history of EC in any first-degree relative.

This model considers only CRC patients as probands and its utility has been analyzed considering EC instead. It is based on the data from CRC patients under 55 years of the publication.

MMRpro model [25] uses the following variables for the proband and first - and second-degree relatives: ages at diagnosis of colorectal and ECs and current age or age at last follow-up for those unaffected by CRC or EC. A meta-analysis involving population-based studies was used to develop this model.

Limitations: As we have highlighted, the three models including different items (Table 6), are based either on population based registries, Myriad data or specific high-risk registries information and different numbers have been used in cohort derivation and in validation tool development.

Performance comparisons of all three were done to see whether they could predict the probability of carrying a Germline mutation of the three studied genes in CRC [26] and EC [27].

In the study by Mercado et al. where 3% of population based EC had LS $PREMM_{1,2,6}$, MMRpredict, and MMRpro were able to distinguish mutation carriers from non-carriers with the area under a receiver operating curve (AUC) of 0.77, 0.76, and 0.77, respectively.

Table 5. Web pages to access Models to predict carrier probabilities in LS

$PREMM_{1,2,6}$ model: http://premm.dfci.harvard.edu/
MMR predict: http://hnpccpredict.hgu.mrc.ac.uk/
MMRPro: CaGene software available free with registration: http://www4.utsouthwestern.edu/breasthealth/cagene/

Table 6. Comparison of predictive models for LS with a focus on EC

Predictive Model	Derivation +Validation Cohort	Genes included	EC index case	Other LS cancers than CRC and EC included	First degree EC included	Synchronicity Index case
$PREMM_{1,2,6,}$	4538+1827	MLH1, MSH2, MSH6	Yes	Yes	Yes	Yes (all LS related cancers)
MMRPredict	870+155	MLH1, MSH2, MSH6	No	No	Yes	Yes (only EC and CRC)
MMRPro	N/A+144	MLH1, MSH2, MSH6	Yes	No	Yes	Yes (only EC and CRC)

Regarding sensitivity and specificity, $PREMM_{1,2,6}$, had 93% and 5%, MMRpredict, 71% and 64% and MMRpro, 57% and 85%. They observed that among mutation carriers 77% had MSI-H tumors and 94% had loss of MMR proteins. They conclude that these predictive models have low clinical utility in selecting EC patients for further testing and recommend the use of IHC and MSI testing.

Of note, none of them include prediction for carrying a Germline mutation in*PMS2* nor *EPCAM*.

Pathologic Identification Criteria

Revised Bethesda criteria [10] (table 2) have since its publication in 2004 included some pathologic features of CRC associated to LS. Some histopathologic features (table 7) have been described that can also prompt suspicion of LS.

Tumor Type

Several studies have shown that there is a wide variety of cell types and similar to the general population [22, 28] while others suggest a higher incidence of non endometrioid type [29, 30]. The median age at LS diagnosis is 46.4 years compared to the general population with 65 to 68 years [31].

Lower Uterine Segment

The lower uterine segment location is found [32] in 3.5% of EC cases and is associated to younger age (54.2 v 62.9 years, p=0.001). In this study, the prevalence of LS in this selected population was as high as 14% when a germ-line mutation of MMR genes was identified and 29% (95% CI, 16.0% to 45.0%) had MMR IHC loss. Another study [14] by Garg showed a higher rate of tumor in this location in EC patients with loss of MMR protein expression.

We have to keep in mind that differential diagnosis with cervical adenocarcinoma through Magnetic Resonance (MRI [33]), IHC [31] or HPV testing [34] may represent a problem.

Lymphocitic Infiltration and Dedifferentiation

In the aforementioned Garg study [14] EC with loss of MMR protein expression was associated to higher lymphocitic infiltration and dedifferentiation compared to those without protein loss.

In a cohort study, LS was known to be associated to EC and 42% of them had at least one of the four pathologic features [22] shown in table 7.

Nevertheless dedifferentiation showed low reproducibility as suggested elsewhere [35]. On the contrary, lymphocitic infiltration showed no correlation with MSI in another study [36].

Table 7. Cardinal pathologic features of LS-associated EC

Lower uterine segment
peritumoral lymphocytes visible at scanning magnification
tumor-infiltrating lymphocytes (TILs): 40 per 10 high-power fields
tumor heterogeneity (specifically, the presence of dedifferentiated carcinoma)

Limitations

The College of American Pathologists has released a statement [37] suggesting that pathologists "need to recognize the histologic and clinical features that should prompt at least a recommendation for MMR" that is focused on colorectal carcinoma.

In spite of this, pathologic features of LS-related EC are not as well-defined [20] and mainly endometrial-type are reported. Moreover sensitivity remains poor and some show contradictory results.

Molecular Models for Prediction and Identification

As previously mentioned, LS is caused by germline mutations in one of the four DNA mismatch repair (MMR) genes: *MLH1*, *MSH2*, *MSH6* and *PMS2*. It has recently been shown that a small proportion of LS patients harbour germline deletions involving the 3'exon of *EPCAM* (*TACSTD1*), a non-MMR gene, that lead to inactivation of the *MSH2* gene via promoter hypermethylation [38, 39]. The biological relevance of germline mutations in other LS related genes such as *MLH3*, *MSH3*, *EXO1*, *PMS1*, or *TGFBR2* has not yet been determined [40-43]. Hence, the definitive test to help identify LS includes performing a mutation analysis of MMR genes, a previous screening on tumor samples including immunohistochemistry (IHC), microsatellite instability (MSI) and *MLH1* promoter methylation analysis in order to identify individuals with a high probability of carrying a germline mutation.

Molecular Screening: Tumor Analysis

1. Microsatellite Instability Analysis

DNA MMR system defects resulted in a mutated phenotype. These mutations accumulate more frequently in short repetitive DNA sequences (micro-satellites). Therefore, MSI analysis comparing a specific microsatellite markers panel using tumor-isolated DNA *versus* DNA from normal tissue or blood can be used as an indication of a possible MMR defect. The most widely accepted microsatellite marker panel is the one recommended by the National Cancer Institute (NCI) with five markers (Bethesda markers): two mono-nucleotide (*BAT25* and *BAT26*) and three dinucleotide markers (*D5S346*, *D2S 123* and *D17S250*) [44].

However, the inclusion of three dinucleotide markers has been questioned because they are less sensitive and specific than mononucleotide repeats for identifying MMR deficiencies.

Table 8. Interpretation of MSI results

Tumor	MSI results
MSI-high (MSI-H)	Instability at >30% of the markers
MSI-low (MSI-L)	Instability at <30% of the markers
MSI-stable (MSS)	No instability

In fact, several microsatellite panels including exclusively quasi-monomorphic mononucleotide markers have been proposed and compared with the one from NCI [45-49]. These panels also have the advantage that the MSI analysis can be assessed without the need for corresponding germline DNA matching [45, 49].

As result of a MSI analysis, tumors can be classified as MSI-H, MSI-L and MSS as shown on table 8 [44].

Those tumors with MSI-H are then analyzed for: *MLH1* promoter methylation or directly MMR gene sequencing, depending on the IHC results.

However, cases with *MSH6* mutation cases are generally associated to MSI-L or MSS and represent an exception.

In a large unselected EC cohort Mercado et al. [27] described a MSI frequency of 23% (19% MSI-H and 4% MSI-L). A relevant observation in this series is that 15% (2) and 8% (1) of the 13 mutation carriers in whom they performed a MSI analysis presented MSI-L and a MSS respectively, all corresponding to *MSH6* mutation carriers. On the other hand, *MLH1* and *MSH 2* mutation carriers had MSI-H tumors [27].

In conclusion, abnormal MSI had 92% sensitivity and 78% specificity for identifying LS (PPV of 9% and NPV of 99.8%) [27]. Similarly, Ryan et al. [22] identified that 2 out of 20 (10%) LS women presenting EC had MSI-S tumors, corresponding to *MSH2* and *MSH6* mutation carriers, and concluded that the sensitivity of MSI testing is only 77% for *MSH6* mutations compared with 89% for *MLH1* and *MSH2* mutations, depending on the number of mononucleotide markers examined. Given the high rate of *MSH2* and *MSH6* germline mutations in EC patients associated with LS, an accurate IHC screening is crucial in these cases.

2. Immunohistochemistry for MMR Proteins (table 9)

MMR gene defect leads to the corresponding loss of protein expression.

Hence, the IHC analyses of the four MMR proteins can be used to identify the mutated gene. MLH1 and PMS2 proteins and MSH2 and MSH6 form functional heterodimers, MLH1 and MSH2 being the mandatory partners of each dimmer, and then testing for specific IHC patterns:

Table 9. Patterns of IHC according to mutated genotype

	MLH1 expression	MSH2 expression	MSH6 expression	PMS2 expression
Mutation or methylation of *MLH1*	lost	conserved	conserved	lost
MSH2 mutation or partial *EPCAM* deletion	conserved	lost	lost	conserved
PMS2 mutation	conserved	conserved	conserved	lost
MSH6 mutation	conserved	conserved	lost	conserved

IHC is an available, simple and inexpensive procedure that can also direct the mutation analysis to a specific MMR gene. By contrast, this technique presents other disadvantages derived from the quality of tissue preparation and the subjective and difficult interpretation of the staining that requires a complete loss of nuclear staining with an internal positive control, especially concerning MSH6. Mercado et al. [27] concluded in their unselected EC cohort that abnormal IHC was consistent with gene mutation with a sensitivity and specificity of 86% and 67% respectively (PPV of 10%, and NPV of 99%). Previously, Lu et al. [16] in their study of women with EC diagnosed under 50 years reported that IHC for MLH1, MSH2 and MSH6 had a sensitivity of 11%, 78% and 67% and a specificity of 86%, 93% and 93% respectively for detecting a germline mutation (does not include *EPCAM* testing).

3. *MLH1* Promoter Methylation Analysis and *BRAF* V600E Mutation

Approximately 20% of sporadic ECs exhibit MSI due to somatic hypermethylation of *MLH1* promoter and consequent transcriptional silencing of the gene [50, 51]. In these cases, MSI is also accompanied by protein loss.

Hence, a molecular test to detect *MLH1* hypermethylation is mandatory in order to identify these sporadic tumors. However, it should be taken into account that constitutional promoter methylation of *MLH1* has recently been reported to be associated with LS and should also be included in LS screening when hypermethylation is detected in tumor [52-54].

Somatic *BRAF* V600E mutation analysis is also included in general LS screening algorithm in order to identify sporadic tumors in colorectal tumors with loss of MLH1expression. Nevertheless, there is controversy over the usefulness of *BRAF* V600E screening in EC [55, 56]. In fact, several studies revealed a very low rate of this mutation in EC [57-60], although some authors have reported that up to 41% of ECs with MSI-H also carried *BRAF* mutation [61].

Germline Mutation Analysis

Tumors with MSI-H and loss of any of the MMR proteins, excluding cases with *MLH1* methylation, are likely to be LS. In these patients, the confirmatory step is to perform a germline mutation analysis of the potentially altered genes based on IHC patterns, using DNA from peripheral blood. The gold standard technique for point mutation detection is direct sequencing of the whole coding sequence and intron-exon boundaries of each gene. Once a point mutation is excluded, large genomic rearrangements (LGRs) (deletions and insertions) must also be analysed, mainly by MLPA (Multiplex ligation-dependent probe amplification). LGRs were present in a relatively high incidence (10-20%) among LS families depending on the clinical criteria used for family selection and on the methodology employed [62].

The gene most frequently affected by LGRs is *MSH2,* mainly as a consequence of Alu-Alu sequence recombination. As previously mentioned, patients with protein loss of MSH2 and MSI-H with no genetic alterations of *MSH2* must also be tested for germline *EPCAM* deletions [38, 39].

Among EC associated to LS, the mutation rate for *MSH2* is 50-66%, followed by *MLH1* with a frequency of 24-40% and *MSH6* (10-13%) [63]; *PMS2* mutations represent <5%. In a prospective series of 100 women with EC diagnosed at age younger than 50 years, Lu et al. [16] identified nine mutation carriers: one (11%) in *MLH1*, 7 (78%) in *MSH2* and one (11%) in *MSH6.* However, Mercado et al. [27] in their cohort of 563 unselected EC cases identified a total of 14 (2.5%) pathogenic mutations: 2 (14%) in *MLH1*, 3 (21%) in *MSH2* and 9 (64%) in *MSH6.*

Clinical Implications

Cumulative Risks

Early reports of cumulative lifetime risks of endometrial and colorectal carcinoma have probably overestimated the figures because patients were identified based on the family cancer history, Therefore ascertainment bias needs to be taken into account in retrospective studies. A woman with LS has a lifetime risk [64, 65] of EC of 42-60% compared to 30-54% of risk of CRC by age 70. When correction for the size of the families ascertained was implemented, lifetime risk in women for EC and CRC were respectively 31.5% and 26.7% [66]. Women with LS are diagnosed with EC at a median age of 48 years [27-72], 57% of cases occurring <50 years of age [67], 61% have a second primary tumor and 15% have more than two tumors.

A recent study [68] of secondary malignancies in women with EC-LS following 20 years reported risks of CRC (48%, 95% confidence interval [CI] = 35% to 62%), cancer of the kidney, renal pelvis, or ureter (11%, 95% CI = 3% to 20%); urinary bladder cancer (9%, 95% CI = 2% to 17%); and breast cancer (11%, 95% CI = 4% to 19%).

Genotype-Phenotype Correlation

Furthermore, recent advances have not included penetrance estimates of *MLH1* and *MSH2* but also on *MSH6*, *PMS2* and *EPCAM*. Genotype-phenotype correlations specifically of relevance to identification, surveillance and management issues, have been identified.

We will summarize penetrance estimates for the two most frequent LS associated cancers in carriers of Germline mutations in *MLH1*, *MSH2* [63, 69], *MSH6*, *PMS2* [70] and *EPCAM* [71] in Table 9.

If we use the identification criteria of less than 50 years we will miss most MSH6 carriers with either CRC or EC as index cases and we may not identify PMS2 associated LS.

Survival

MSI has emerged as an independent prognostic factor of survival in some series but there are striking differences between methods for defining MSI-H tumors with either one marker, IHC staining of MMRProteins and scarce use of the complete 5 MSI panel proposed by the NCI (table 10). The possible interpretation of these disparities may lay in the fact that across studies there is a diversity of stage I tumors and histologic subtypes while adjuvant treatment is not always reported or consistent [36, 72-78].

Table 9. Genotype-phenotype correlation in LS

	CRC estimates at 70 years (%)	Median age CRC	EC estimates at 70 years (%)	median age EC
General population	**5,5**	**68**	**2,7**	**61**
MLH1	41-53	45	32-54	49
MSH2	39-48	44	21-44	48
MSH6	10-12	54	16-26	55
PMS2	15-20	61-66	15	49
EPCAM	75	43	12	49

Table 10. Selected studies in EC with prognostic value of MSI

Author	Journal	Year	N	MSI-H (%)	Selected cases	MSI definition in the study	Association	OS
Honore	2006	Int. J. Gynecol. Cancer	218	16	Endometroid EC	BAT26	Grade	Not directly explored; correlates with aggressive features
							Endometrial atrophy	
							Squamous metaplasia	
							Isthmic involvement	
							Depth of myoinvasion	
							Vascular invasion	
							Extrauterine and extramy ometrial spread	
Arabi	2009	Gynecol. Oncol.	119		High Grade EC	IHC loss: MLH1, MSH2, MSH6		Median survival 3 months vs 71 months, p=0.04
Mackay	2010	Eur. J. Cancer	163	19	EC	BAT25+Bat26		Not improved OS HR 0.67, 95% CI 0.34-1.33; p=0.25
								In early stage I/II HR 0.06 95% CI 0.05-0.50; p<0.0001 for overall survival

Author	Journal	Year	N	MSI-H (%)	Selected cases	MSI definition in the study	Association	OS
An	2007	Am. J. Surg. Pathol.	100	18	EC	NCI Panel	Lymphovascular invasion	Not explored; correlates with aggressive features
							Deep myometrial invasion	
							Higher clinical stages	
Zighelboim	2007	J. Clin. Oncol.	446	33	Endometroid EC	NCI Panel	Higher stage	N HR1,011 [0.688 to 1.484]
							Grade	
Black	2006	J. Clin. Oncol.	473	20	EC	NCI Panel	Higher stage	DFS HR 0.3 [0.4-0.7]
							myometrial invasion	
Bilbao	2010	Int. J. Radat. Oncol. Biol. Phys.	93	22	EC treated with RT	BAT25 BAT26 NR21 NR24 NR27	Higher stage	Not in whole series
							Higher grade	In early stages DFS HR 3.25 [1.01-10.49]
Steinbakk	2011	Mod. Pathol.	224	15	FIGO I Endometroid EC	BAT25 BAT26 NR21 NR24 NR27		MSI-H worse survival

In a recent metaanalysis [79] no significant association between MMR deficiency and worse OS (6 studies, hazard ratio [HR] 2.0, $p = 0.11$) or DFS (4 studies, HR ratio 1.31, $p = 0.66$) was observed. Moreover, no potential prognostic value of mutational status of germline MMR genes in EC was observed [80]. Risk reduction strategies for gynecologic cancer in LS

Screening Procedures for EC

Efficacy of cancer screening procedures is defined by the ability to detect precursors and remove them before cancer occurs, thus increasing overall survival. This seems to be the case for CRC screening with colonoscopy in LS. Nevertheless, efficacy of screening women at risk of EC and ovarian cancer in LS patients is still controversial and lacks good levels of evidence.

In 25 prophylactic hysterectomies in LS patients, 24% presented endometrium abnormalities, 12% atypical complex hyperplasia, 8% endometrial carcinoma above 50 years of age and 4% simple hyperplasia [81]. Lesions were focal and this could explain difficulty in early detection despite curettage [82]. This tumorigenic mechanism via complex hyperplasia with or without atypia has been observed elsewhere [83] nevertheless molecular genetics alterations were observed years before cancer. A systematic review [84] of 647 women with LS undergoing surveillance for EC with ultrasound (2 studies), ultrasound and endometrial biopsy (2 studies) or endometrial biopsy (one study) showed that the ultrasound only modality detected no EC and only interval cancers were observed whereas approaches that included biopsy improved the detection of precursor lesions or EC.

In theory, one of the benefits of EC screening is early detection which is addressed in this study [85]. They reported more cases of EC with screening procedures compared with waiting for symptoms to appear, despite the lack of statistical significance.

The value of surveillance is still unknown but guidelines [86, 87] based on expert consensus recommend gynaecological examination, transvaginal ultrasound and aspiration biopsy starting between the ages of 35–40 years.

If endometrial sampling is performed at the moment of colonoscopy it is generally more acceptable to patients [88].

Current recommendations do not include the information provided by genotype-phenotype correlation into clinical practice.

Prophylactic Surgery

Total Histerectomy and bilateral salpingoophorectomy (TAH-BSO) was shown to significantly reduce the risk of endometrial cancer in women with

Lynch syndrome [89] as well as a risk for ovarian cancer. It has proven to be the most cost effective approach in gynecologic malignancies in LS [90].

Guidelines [86, 87] suggest that the option of prophylactic hysterectomy should be discussed with mutation carriers who have completed their family and TAH is best done at the moment of colon surgery. The optimal timing should be around 40 years of age; there is no agreement about BSO in premenopausal women because of the lower risk of ovarian cancer.

Conclusion

As LS is an evolving field with novelties occurring in identification criteria, molecular basis and clinical management a comprehensive approach should be implemented at all levels.

There is a general understanding among Genetic Counselors that LS is difficult to identify among EC patients with current consensus clinical criteria. A so-called universal approach that includes either IHC and/or MSI in all EC patients has been advocated and is currently being used among 50% of centers in a survey [91]. When considering not only the detection rate but cost, IHC triage of women with EC at any age having at least 1 first-degree relative with an LS-associated cancer seems a cost-effective strategy for detecting LS [92].

A body of knowledge has been developing recently to include genotype-phenotype correlations that might be relevant to identification, molecular studies and clinical management.

So far these nuances have not modified guidelines and are slowly reaching the clinic. As an example EPCAM loss resulting in MSH2 disfunction seems to have new implications for molecular study and different penetrance than MSH2 mutation carriers.

Although level of evidence for clinical management of EC-LS is low we must adhere to guidelines and share the evidence with members at risk to help select the prevention options.

References

[1] Dinh, T. A., Rosner, B. I., Atwood, J. C., Boland, C. R., Syngal, S., Vasen, H. F., Gruber, S. B., Burt, R. W. Health benefits and cost-

effectiveness of primary genetic screening for Lynch syndrome in the general population. *Cancer Prev. Res.* (Phila.) 4: 9-22.

[2] Eng, C. Will the real Cowden syndrome please stand up: revised diagnostic criteria. *J. Med. Genet.* 12000;37: 828-30.

[3] Ni, Y., Zbuk, K. M., Sadler, T., Patocs, A., Lobo, G., Edelman, E., Platzer, P., Orloff, M. S., Waite, K. A., Eng, C. Germline mutations and variants in the succinate dehydrogenase genes in Cowden and Cowden-like syndromes. *Am. J. Hum. Genet.* 12008;83: 261-8.

[4] Li, F. P., Fraumeni, J. F., Jr., Mulvihill, J. J., Blattner, W. A., Dreyfus, M. G., Tucker, M. A., Miller, R. W. A cancer family syndrome in twenty-four kindreds. *Cancer Res.* 11988;48: 5358-62.

[5] Pennington, K. P., Walsh, T., Lee, M., Pennil, C., Novetsky, A. P., Agnew, K. J., Thornton, A., Garcia, R., Mutch, D., King, M. C., Goodfellow, P., Swisher, E. M. BRCA1, TP53, and CHEK2 germline mutations in uterine serous carcinoma. *Cancer* 119: 332-8.

[6] Lynch, H. T., de la Chapelle, A. Hereditary colorectal cancer. *N. Engl. J. Med.* 12003;348: 919-32.

[7] Weissman, S. M., Burt, R., Church, J., Erdman, S., Hampel, H., Holter, S., Jasperson, K., Kalady, M. F., Haidle, J. L., Lynch, H. T., Palaniappan, S., Wise, P. E., Senter, L. Identification of individuals at risk for Lynch syndrome using targeted evaluations and genetic testing: National Society of Genetic Counselors and the Collaborative Group of the Americas on Inherited Colorectal Cancer joint practice guideline. *J. Genet. Couns.* 21: 484-93.

[8] Lu, K. H., Dinh, M., Kohlmann, W., Watson, P., Green, J., Syngal, S., Bandipalliam, P., Chen, L. M., Allen, B., Conrad, P., Terdiman, J., Sun, C., Daniels, M., Burke, T., Gershenson, D. M., Lynch, H., Lynch, P., Broaddus, R. R. Gynecologic cancer as a "sentinel cancer" for women with hereditary nonpolyposis colorectal cancer syndrome. *Obstet. Gynecol.* 12005;105: 569-74.

[9] Vasen, H. F., Watson, P., Mecklin, J. P., Lynch, H. T. New clinical criteria for hereditary nonpolyposis colorectal cancer (HNPCC, Lynch syndrome) proposed by the International Collaborative group on HNPCC. *Gastroenterology* 11999;116: 1453-6.

[10] Umar, A., Boland, C. R., Terdiman, J. P., Syngal, S., de la Chapelle, A., Ruschoff, J., Fishel, R., Lindor, N. M., Burgart, L. J., Hamelin, R., Hamilton, S. R., Hiatt, R. A., Jass, J., Lindblom, A., Lynch, H. T., Peltomaki, P., Ramsey, S. D., Rodriguez-Bigas, M. A., Vasen, H. F., Hawk, E. T., Barrett, J. C., Freedman, A. N., Srivastava, S. Revised

Bethesda Guidelines for hereditary nonpolyposis colorectal cancer (Lynch syndrome) and microsatellite instability. *J. Natl. Cancer Inst.* l2004;96: 261-8.

[11] Lancaster, J. M., Powell, C. B., Kauff, N. D., Cass, I., Chen, L. M., Lu, K. H., Mutch, D. G., Berchuck, A., Karlan, B. Y., Herzog, T. J. Society of Gynecologic Oncologists Education Committee statement on risk assessment for inherited gynecologic cancer predispositions. *Gynecol. Oncol.* l2007;107: 159-62.

[12] Soliman, P. T., Broaddus, R. R., Schmeler, K. M., Daniels, M. S., Gonzalez, D., Slomovitz, B. M., Gershenson, D. M., Lu, K. H. Women with synchronous primary cancers of the endometrium and ovary: do they have Lynch syndrome? *J. Clin. Oncol.* l2005;23: 9344-50.

[13] Kim, M. K., Song, S. Y., Do, I. G., Kim, S. H., Choi, C. H., Kim, T. J., Lee, J. W., Bae, D. S., Kim, B. G. Synchronous gynecologic malignancy and preliminary results of Lynch syndrome. *J. Gynecol. Oncol.* 22: 233-8.

[14] Garg, K., Leitao, M. M., Jr., Kauff, N. D., Hansen, J., Kosarin, K., Shia, J., Soslow, R. A. Selection of endometrial carcinomas for DNA mismatch repair protein immunohistochemistry using patient age and tumor morphology enhances detection of mismatch repair abnormalities. *Am. J. Surg. Pathol.* l2009;33: 925-33.

[15] Berends, M. J., Wu, Y., Sijmons, R. H., van der Sluis, T., Ek, W. B., Ligtenberg, M. J., Arts, N. J., ten Hoor, K. A., Kleibeuker, J. H., de Vries, E. G., Mourits, M. J., Hollema, H., Buys, C. H., Hofstra, R. M., van der Zee, A. G. Toward new strategies to select young endometrial cancer patients for mismatch repair gene mutation analysis. *J. Clin. Oncol.* l2003;21: 4364-70.

[16] Lu, K. H., Schorge, J. O., Rodabaugh, K. J., Daniels, M. S., Sun, C. C., Soliman, P. T., White, K. G., Luthra, R., Gershenson, D. M., Broaddus, R. R. Prospective determination of prevalence of lynch syndrome in young women with endometrial cancer. *J. Clin. Oncol.* l2007;25: 5158-64.

[17] Win, A. K., Dowty, J. G., Antill, Y. C., English, D. R., Baron, J. A., Young, J. P., Giles, G. G., Southey, M. C., Winship, I., Lipton, L., Parry, S., Thibodeau, S. N., Haile, R. W., Gallinger, S., Le Marchand, L., Lindor, N. M., Newcomb, P. A., Hopper, J. L., Jenkins, M. A. Body mass index in early adulthood and endometrial cancer risk for mismatch repair gene mutation carriers. *Obstet. Gynecol.* 117: 899-905.

[18] Shih, K. K., Garg, K., Levine, D. A., Kauff, N. D., Abu-Rustum, N. R., Soslow, R. A., Barakat, R. R. Clinicopathologic significance of DNA mismatch repair protein defects and endometrial cancer in women 40 years of age and younger. *Gynecol. Oncol.* 123: 88-94.

[19] Hampel, H., Frankel, W., Panescu, J., Lockman, J., Sotamaa, K., Fix, D., Comeras, I., La Jeunesse, J., Nakagawa, H., Westman, J. A., Prior, T. W., Clendenning, M., Penzone, P., Lombardi, J., Dunn, P., Cohn, D. E., Copeland, L., Eaton, L., Fowler, J., Lewandowski, G., Vaccarello, L., Bell, J., Reid, G., de la Chapelle, A. Screening for Lynch syndrome (hereditary nonpolyposis colorectal cancer) among endometrial cancer patients. *Cancer Res.* l2006;66: 7810-7.

[20] Clarke, B. A., Cooper, K. Identifying Lynch syndrome in patients with endometrial carcinoma: shortcomings of morphologic and clinical schemas. *Adv. Anat. Pathol.* 19: 231-8.

[21] Tan, Y. Y., McGaughran, J., Ferguson, K., Walsh, M. D., Buchanan, D. D., Young, J. P., Webb, P. M., Obermair, A., Spurdle, A. B. Improving identification of lynch syndrome patients: a comparison of research data with clinical records. *Int. J. Cancer* 132: 2876-83.

[22] Ryan, P., Mulligan, A. M., Aronson, M., Ferguson, S. E., Bapat, B., Semotiuk, K., Holter, S., Kwon, J., Kalloger, S. E., Gilks, C. B., Gallinger, S., Pollett, A., Clarke, B. A. Comparison of clinical schemas and morphologic features in predicting Lynch syndrome in mutation-positive patients with endometrial cancer encountered in the context of familial gastrointestinal cancer registries. *Cancer* 118: 681-8.

[23] Kastrinos, F., Steyerberg, E. W., Mercado, R., Balmana, J., Holter, S., Gallinger, S., Siegmund, K. D., Church, J. M., Jenkins, M. A., Lindor, N. M., Thibodeau, S. N., Burbidge, L. A., Wenstrup, R. J., Syngal, S. The PREMM(1,2,6) model predicts risk of MLH1, MSH2, and MSH6 germline mutations based on cancer history. *Gastroenterology* 140: 73-81.

[24] Barnetson, R. A., Tenesa, A., Farrington, S. M., Nicholl, I. D., Cetnarskyj, R., Porteous, M. E., Campbell, H., Dunlop, M. G. Identification and survival of carriers of mutations in DNA mismatch-repair genes in colon cancer. *N. Engl. J. Med.* l2006;354: 2751-63.

[25] Chen, S., Wang, W., Lee, S., Nafa, K., Lee, J., Romans, K., Watson, P., Gruber, S. B., Euhus, D., Kinzler, K. W., Jass, J., Gallinger, S., Lindor, N. M., Casey, G., Ellis, N., Giardiello, F. M., Offit, K., Parmigiani, G. Prediction of germline mutations and cancer risk in the Lynch syndrome. *JAMA* l2006;296: 1479-87.

[26] Pouchet, C. J., Wong, N., Chong, G., Sheehan, M. J., Schneider, G., Rosen-Sheidley, B., Foulkes, W., Tischkowitz, M. A comparison of models used to predict MLH1, MSH2 and MSH6 mutation carriers. *Ann. Oncol.* l2009;20: 681-8.

[27] Mercado, R. C., Hampel, H., Kastrinos, F., Steyerberg, E., Balmana, J., Stoffel, E., Cohn, D. E., Backes, F. J., Hopper, J. L., Jenkins, M. A., Lindor, N. M., Casey, G., Haile, R., Madhavan, S., de la Chapelle, A., Syngal, S. Performance of PREMM(1,2,6), MMRpredict, and MMRpro in detecting Lynch syndrome among endometrial cancer cases. *Genet. Med.* 14: 670-80.

[28] Broaddus, R. R., Lynch, H. T., Chen, L. M., Daniels, M. S., Conrad, P., Munsell, M. F., White, K. G., Luthra, R., Lu, K. H. Pathologic features of endometrial carcinoma associated with HNPCC: a comparison with sporadic endometrial carcinoma. *Cancer* l2006;106: 87-94.

[29] Carcangiu, M. L., Radice, P., Casalini, P., Bertario, L., Merola, M., Sala, P. Lynch syndrome--related endometrial carcinomas show a high frequency of nonendometrioid types and of high FIGO grade endometrioid types. *Int. J. Surg. Pathol.* 18: 21-6.

[30] Palacios, J. A. C., Lujan, D., et al. Pathological features of endometrial cancer in patients with Lynch syndrome. *Lab. Invest.* l2010;90: 258A.

[31] Djordjevic, B., Westin, S., Broaddus, R. R. Application of Immunohistochemistry and Molecular Diagnostics to Clinically Relevant Problems in Endometrial Cancer Bojana Djordjevic, Shannon Westin, Russell R. Broaddus. *Surg. Pathol. Clin.* 5: 859-878.

[32] Westin, S. N., Lacour, R. A., Urbauer, D. L., Luthra, R., Bodurka, D. C., Lu, K. H., Broaddus, R. R. Carcinoma of the lower uterine segment: a newly described association with Lynch syndrome. *J. Clin. Oncol.* l2008;26: 5965-71.

[33] Haider, M. A., Patlas, M., Jhaveri, K., Chapman, W., Fyles, A., Rosen, B. Adenocarcinoma involving the uterine cervix: magnetic resonance imaging findings in tumours of endometrial, compared with cervical, origin. *Can. Assoc. Radiol. J.* l2006;57: 43-8.

[34] Ansari-Lari, M. A., Staebler, A., Zaino, R. J., Shah, K. V., Ronnett, B. M. Distinction of endocervical and endometrial adenocarcinomas: immunohistochemical p16 expression correlated with human papillomavirus (HPV) DNA detection. *Am. J. Surg. Pathol.* l2004;28: 160-7.

[35] Tafe, L. J., Garg, K., Chew, I., Tornos, C., Soslow, R. A. Endometrial and ovarian carcinomas with undifferentiated components: clinically

aggressive and frequently underrecognized neoplasms. *Mod. Pathol.* 23: 781-9.

[36] Honore, L. H., Hanson, J., Andrew, S. E. Microsatellite instability in endometrioid endometrial carcinoma: correlation with clinically relevant pathologic variables. *Int. J. Gynecol. Cancer* l2006;16: 1386-92.

[37] Turner, J. W. F. L., Bloom, K. J., et al. Prognostic uses of MSI testing 2011. In: http://www.cap.org/apps/docs/committees/technology/micro satellite_testing.pdf.

[38] Kuiper, R. P., Vissers, L. E., Venkatachalam, R., Bodmer, D., Hoenselaar, E., Goossens, M., Haufe, A., Kamping, E., Niessen, R. C., Hogervorst, F. B., Gille, J. J., Redeker, B., Tops, C. M., van Gijn, M. E., van den Ouweland, A. M., Rahner, N., Steinke, V., Kahl, P., Holinski-Feder, E., Morak, M., Kloor, M., Stemmler, S., Betz, B., Hutter, P., Bunyan, D. J., Syngal, S., Culver, J. O., Graham, T., Chan, T. L., Nagtegaal, I. D., van Krieken, J. H., Schackert, H. K., Hoogerbrugge, N., van Kessel, A. G., Ligtenberg, M. J. Recurrence and variability of germline EPCAM deletions in Lynch syndrome. *Hum. Mutat.* 32: 407-14.

[39] Ligtenberg, M. J., Kuiper, R. P., Chan, T. L., Goossens, M., Hebeda, K. M., Voorendt, M., Lee, T. Y., Bodmer, D., Hoenselaar, E., Hendriks-Cornelissen, S. J., Tsui, W. Y., Kong, C. K., Brunner, H. G., van Kessel, A. G., Yuen, S. T., van Krieken, J. H., Leung, S. Y., Hoogerbrugge, N. Heritable somatic methylation and inactivation of MSH2 in families with Lynch syndrome due to deletion of the 3' exons of TACSTD1. *Nat. Genet.* l2009;41: 112-7.

[40] Wu, Y., Berends, M. J., Post, J. G., Mensink, R. G., Verlind, E., Van Der Sluis, T., Kempinga, C., Sijmons, R. H., van der Zee, A. G., Hollema, H., Kleibeuker, J. H., Buys, C. H., Hofstra, R. M. Germline mutations of EXO1 gene in patients with hereditary nonpolyposis colorectal cancer (HNPCC) and atypical HNPCC forms. *Gastroenterology* l2001;120: 1580-7.

[41] Lu, S. L., Kawabata, M., Imamura, T., Akiyama, Y., Nomizu, T., Miyazono, K., Yuasa, Y. HNPCC associated with germline mutation in the TGF-beta type II receptor gene. *Nat. Genet.* l1998;19: 17-8.

[42] Peltomaki, P. Role of DNA mismatch repair defects in the pathogenesis of human cancer. *J. Clin. Oncol.* l2003;21: 1174-9.

[43] Liu, H. X., Zhou, X. L., Liu, T., Werelius, B., Lindmark, G., Dahl, N., Lindblom, A. The role of hMLH3 in familial colorectal cancer. *Cancer Res.* l2003;63: 1894-9.

[44] Boland, C. R., Thibodeau, S. N., Hamilton, S. R., Sidransky, D., Eshleman, J. R., Burt, R. W., Meltzer, S. J., Rodriguez-Bigas, M. A., Fodde, R., Ranzani, G. N., Srivastava, S. A National Cancer Institute Workshop on Microsatellite Instability for cancer detection and familial predisposition: development of international criteria for the determination of microsatellite instability in colorectal cancer. *Cancer Res.* 11998; 58: 5248-57.

[45] Xicola, R. M., Llor, X., Pons, E., Castells, A., Alenda, C., Pinol, V., Andreu, M., Castellvi-Bel, S., Paya, A., Jover, R., Bessa, X., Giros, A., Duque, J. M., Nicolas-Perez, D., Garcia, A. M., Rigau, J., Gassull, M. A. Performance of different microsatellite marker panels for detection of mismatch repair-deficient colorectal tumors. *J. Natl. Cancer Inst.* 12007; 99: 244-52.

[46] Suraweera, N., Duval, A., Reperant, M., Vaury, C., Furlan, D., Leroy, K., Seruca, R., Iacopetta, B., Hamelin, R. Evaluation of tumor microsatellite instability using five quasimonomorphic mononucleotide repeats and pentaplex PCR. *Gastroenterology* 12002;123: 1804-11.

[47] Bacher, J. W., Flanagan, L. A., Smalley, R. L., Nassif, N. A., Burgart, L. J., Halberg, R. B., Megid, W. M., Thibodeau, S. N. Development of a fluorescent multiplex assay for detection of MSI-High tumors. *Dis. Markers* 12004;20: 237-50.

[48] Buhard, O., Suraweera, N., Lectard, A., Duval, A., Hamelin, R. Quasimonomorphic mononucleotide repeats for high-level microsatellite instability analysis. *Dis. Markers* 12004;20: 251-7.

[49] Murphy, K. M., Zhang, S., Geiger, T., Hafez, M. J., Bacher, J., Berg, K. D., Eshleman, J. R. Comparison of the microsatellite instability analysis system and the Bethesda panel for the determination of microsatellite instability in colorectal cancers. *J. Mol. Diagn.* 12006;8: 305-11.

[50] De Leeuw, W. J., Dierssen, J., Vasen, H. F., Wijnen, J. T., Kenter, G. G., Meijers-Heijboer, H., Brocker-Vriends, A., Stormorken, A., Moller, P., Menko, F., Cornelisse, C. J., Morreau, H. Prediction of a mismatch repair gene defect by microsatellite instability and immunohistochemical analysis in endometrial tumours from HNPCC patients. *J. Pathol.* 12000; 192: 328-35.

[51] Bruegl, A. S., Djordjevic, B., Urbauer, D. L., Westin, S. N., Soliman, P. T., Lu, K. H., Luthra, R., Broaddus, R. R. Utility of MLH1 Methylation Analysis in the Clinical Evaluation of Lynch Syndrome in Women with Endometrial Cancer. *Curr. Pharm. Des.*

[52] Ward, R. L., Dobbins, T., Lindor, N. M., Rapkins, R. W., Hitchins, M. P. Identification of constitutional MLH1 epimutations and promoter variants in colorectal cancer patients from the Colon Cancer Family Registry. *Genet. Med.* 15: 25-35.

[53] Hitchins, M. P., Ward, R. L. Constitutional (germline) MLH1 epimutation as an aetiological mechanism for hereditary non-polyposis colorectal cancer. *J. Med. Genet.* l2009;46: 793-802.

[54] Hitchins, M. P., Rapkins, R. W., Kwok, C. T., Srivastava, S., Wong, J. J., Khachigian, L. M., Polly, P., Goldblatt, J., Ward, R. L. Dominantly inherited constitutional epigenetic silencing of MLH1 in a cancer-affected family is linked to a single nucleotide variant within the 5'UTR. *Cancer Cell* 20: 200-13.

[55] Kawaguchi, M., Yanokura, M., Banno, K., Kobayashi, Y., Kuwabara, Y., Kobayashi, M., Nomura, H., Hirasawa, A., Susumu, N., Aoki, D. Analysis of a correlation between the BRAF V600E mutation and abnormal DNA mismatch repair in patients with sporadic endometrial cancer. *Int. J. Oncol.* l2009;34: 1541-7.

[56] He, M., Breese, V., Hang, S., Zhang, C., Xiong, J., Jackson, C. BRAF V600E Mutations in Endometrial Adenocarcinoma. *Diagn. Mol. Pathol.* 22: 35-40.

[57] Mutch, D. G., Powell, M. A., Mallon, M. A., Goodfellow, P. J. RAS/RAF mutation and defective DNA mismatch repair in endometrial cancers. *Am. J. Obstet. Gynecol.* l2004;190: 935-42.

[58] Salvesen, H. B., Kumar, R., Stefansson, I., Angelini, S., MacDonald, N., Smeds, J., Jacobs, I. J., Hemminki, K., Das, S., Akslen, L. A. Low frequency of BRAF and CDKN2A mutations in endometrial cancer. *Int. J. Cancer* l2005;115: 930-4.

[59] Pappa, K. I., Choleza, M., Markaki, S., Giannikaki, E., Kyroudi, A., Vlachos, G., Voulgaris, Z., Anagnou, N. P. Consistent absence of BRAF mutations in cervical and endometrial cancer despite KRAS mutation status. *Gynecol. Oncol.* l2006;100: 596-600.

[60] Peterson, L. M., Kipp, B. R., Halling, K. C., Kerr, S. E., Smith, D. I., Distad, T. J., Clayton, A. C., Medeiros, F. Molecular characterization of endometrial cancer: a correlative study assessing microsatellite instability, MLH1 hypermethylation, DNA mismatch repair protein expression, and PTEN, PIK3CA, KRAS, and BRAF mutation analysis. *Int. J. Gynecol. Pathol.* 31: 195-205.

[61] Feng, Y. Z., Shiozawa, T., Miyamoto, T., Kashima, H., Kurai, M., Suzuki, A., Konishi, I. BRAF mutation in endometrial carcinoma and

hyperplasia: correlation with KRAS and p53 mutations and mismatch repair protein expression. *Clin. Cancer Res.* l2005;11: 6133-8.

[62] Van der Klift, H., Wijnen, J., Wagner, A., Verkuilen, P., Tops, C., Otway, R., Kohonen-Corish, M., Vasen, H., Oliani, C., Barana, D., Moller, P., Delozier-Blanchet, C., Hutter, P., Foulkes, W., Lynch, H., Burn, J., Moslein, G., Fodde, R. Molecular characterization of the spectrum of genomic deletions in the mismatch repair genes MSH2, MLH1, MSH6, and PMS2 responsible for hereditary nonpolyposis colorectal cancer (HNPCC). *Genes Chromosomes Cancer* l2005;44: 123-38.

[63] Bonadona, V., Bonaiti, B., Olschwang, S., Grandjouan, S., Huiart, L., Longy, M., Guimbaud, R., Buecher, B., Bignon, Y. J., Caron, O., Colas, C., Nogues, C., Lejeune-Dumoulin, S., Olivier-Faivre, L., Polycarpe-Osaer, F., Nguyen, T. D., Desseigne, F., Saurin, J. C., Berthet, P., Leroux, D., Duffour, J., Manouvrier, S., Frebourg, T., Sobol, H., Lasset, C., Bonaiti-Pellie, C. Cancer risks associated with germline mutations in MLH1, MSH2, and MSH6 genes in Lynch syndrome. *JAMA* 305: 2304-10.

[64] Aarnio, M., Sankila, R., Pukkala, E., Salovaara, R., Aaltonen, L. A., de la Chapelle, A., Peltomaki, P., Mecklin, J. P., Jarvinen, H. J. Cancer risk in mutation carriers of DNA-mismatch-repair genes. *Int. J. Cancer* l1999; 81: 214-8.

[65] Dunlop, M. G., Farrington, S. M., Carothers, A. D., Wyllie, A. H., Sharp, L., Burn, J., Liu, B., Kinzler, K. W., Vogelstein, B. Cancer risk associated with germline DNA mismatch repair gene mutations. *Hum. Mol. Genet.* l1997;6: 105-10.

[66] Quehenberger, F., Vasen, H. F., van Houwelingen, H. C. Risk of colorectal and endometrial cancer for carriers of mutations of the hMLH1 and hMSH2 gene: correction for ascertainment. *J. Med. Genet.* l2005;42: 491-6.

[67] Vasen, H. F., Watson, P., Mecklin, J. P., Jass, J. R., Green, J. S., Nomizu, T., Muller, H., Lynch, H. T. The epidemiology of endometrial cancer in hereditary nonpolyposis colorectal cancer. *Anticancer Res.* l1994;14: 1675-8.

[68] Win, A. K., Lindor, N. M., Winship, I., Tucker, K. M., Buchanan, D. D., Young, J. P., Rosty, C., Leggett, B., Giles, G. G., Goldblatt, J., Macrae, F. A., Parry, S., Kalady, M. F., Baron, J. A., Ahnen, D. J., Marchand, L. L., Gallinger, S., Haile, R. W., Newcomb, P. A., Hopper, J. L., Jenkins, M. A. Risks of colorectal and other cancers after endometrial cancer for women with Lynch syndrome. *J. Natl. Cancer Inst.* 105: 274-9.

[69] Stoffel, E., Mukherjee, B., Raymond, V. M., Tayob, N., Kastrinos, F., Sparr, J., Wang, F., Bandipalliam, P., Syngal, S., Gruber, S. B. Calculation of risk of colorectal and endometrial cancer among patients with Lynch syndrome. *Gastroenterology* l2009;137: 1621-7.

[70] Senter, L., Clendenning, M., Sotamaa, K., Hampel, H., Green, J., Potter, J. D., Lindblom, A., Lagerstedt, K., Thibodeau, S. N., Lindor, N. M., Young, J., Winship, I., Dowty, J. G., White, D. M., Hopper, J. L., Baglietto, L., Jenkins, M. A., de la Chapelle, A. The clinical phenotype of Lynch syndrome due to germ-line PMS2 mutations. *Gastroenterology* l2008;135: 419-28.

[71] Kempers, M. J., Kuiper, R. P., Ockeloen, C. W., Chappuis, P. O., Hutter, P., Rahner, N., Schackert, H. K., Steinke, V., Holinski-Feder, E., Morak, M., Kloor, M., Buttner, R., Verwiel, E. T., van Krieken, J. H., Nagtegaal, I. D., Goossens, M., van der Post, R. S., Niessen, R. C., Sijmons, R. H., Kluijt, I., Hogervorst, F. B., Leter, E. M., Gille, J. J., Aalfs, C. M., Redeker, E. J., Hes, F. J., Tops, C. M., van Nesselrooij, B. P., van Gijn, M. E., Gomez Garcia, E. B., Eccles, D. M., Bunyan, D. J., Syngal, S., Stoffel, E. M., Culver, J. O., Palomares, M. R., Graham, T., Velsher, L., Papp, J., Olah, E., Chan, T. L., Leung, S. Y., van Kessel, A. G., Kiemeney, L. A., Hoogerbrugge, N., Ligtenberg, M. J. Risk of colorectal and endometrial cancers in EPCAM deletion-positive Lynch syndrome: a cohort study. *Lancet Oncol.* 12: 49-55.

[72] Arabi, H., Guan, H., Kumar, S., Cote, M., Bandyopadhyay, S., Bryant, C., Shah, J., Abdul-Karim, F. W., Munkarah, A. R., Ali-Fehmi, R. Impact of microsatellite instability (MSI) on survival in high grade endometrial carcinoma. *Gynecol. Oncol.* l2009;113: 153-8.

[73] Mackay, H. J., Gallinger, S., Tsao, M. S., McLachlin, C. M., Tu, D., Keiser, K., Eisenhauer, E. A., Oza, A. M. Prognostic value of microsatellite instability (MSI) and PTEN expression in women with endometrial cancer: results from studies of the NCIC Clinical Trials Group (NCIC CTG). *Eur. J. Cancer* 46: 1365-73.

[74] An, H. J., Kim, K. I., Kim, J. Y., Shim, J. Y., Kang, H., Kim, T. H., Kim, J. K., Jeong, J. K., Lee, S. Y., Kim, S. J. Microsatellite instability in endometrioid type endometrial adenocarcinoma is associated with poor prognostic indicators. *Am. J. Surg. Pathol.* l2007;31: 846-53.

[75] Black, D., Soslow, R. A., Levine, D. A., Tornos, C., Chen, S. C., Hummer, A. J., Bogomolniy, F., Olvera, N., Barakat, R. R., Boyd, J. Clinicopathologic significance of defective DNA mismatch repair in endometrial carcinoma. *J. Clin. Oncol.* l2006;24: 1745-53.

[76] Zighelboim, I., Goodfellow, P. J., Gao, F., Gibb, R. K., Powell, M. A., Rader, J. S., Mutch, D. G. Microsatellite instability and epigenetic inactivation of MLH1 and outcome of patients with endometrial carcinomas of the endometrioid type. *J. Clin. Oncol.* l2007;25: 2042-8.

[77] Bilbao, C., Lara, P. C., Ramirez, R., Henriquez-Hernandez, L. A., Rodriguez, G., Falcon, O., Leon, L., Perucho, M., Diaz-Chico, B. N., Diaz-Chico, J. C. Microsatellite instability predicts clinical outcome in radiation-treated endometrioid endometrial cancer. *Int. J. Radiat. Oncol. Biol. Phys.* 76: 9-13.

[78] Steinbakk, A., Malpica, A., Slewa, A., Skaland, I., Gudlaugsson, E., Janssen, E. A., Lovslett, K., Fiane, B., Kruse, A. J., Feng, W., Yinhua, Y., Baak, J. P. Biomarkers and microsatellite instability analysis of curettings can predict the behavior of FIGO stage I endometrial endometrioid adenocarcinoma. *Mod. Pathol.* 24: 1262-71.

[79] Diaz-Padilla, I., Romero, N., Amir, E., Matias-Guiu, X., Vilar, E., Muggia, F., Garcia-Donas, J. Mismatch repair status and clinical outcome in endometrial cancer: A systematic review and meta-analysis. *Crit. Rev. Oncol. Hematol.*

[80] Boks, D. E., Trujillo, A. P., Voogd, A. C., Morreau, H., Kenter, G. G., Vasen, H. F. Survival analysis of endometrial carcinoma associated with hereditary nonpolyposis colorectal cancer. *Int. J. Cancer* l2002;102: 198-200.

[81] Karamurzin, Y., Soslow, R. A., Garg, K. Histologic evaluation of prophylactic hysterectomy and oophorectomy in Lynch syndrome. *Am. J. Surg. Pathol.* 37: 579-85.

[82] Helder-Woolderink, J. M., De Bock, G. H., Sijmons, R. H., Hollema, H., Mourits, M. J. The additional value of endometrial sampling in the early detection of endometrial cancer in women with Lynch syndrome. *Gynecol. Oncol.*

[83] Nieminen, T. T., Gylling, A., Abdel-Rahman, W. M., Nuorva, K., Aarnio, M., Renkonen-Sinisalo, L., Jarvinen, H. J., Mecklin, J. P., Butzow, R., Peltomaki, P. Molecular analysis of endometrial tumorigenesis: importance of complex hyperplasia regardless of atypia. *Clin. Cancer Res.* l2009;15: 5772-83.

[84] Auranen, A., Joutsiniemi, T. A systematic review of gynecological cancer surveillance in women belonging to hereditary nonpolyposis colorectal cancer (Lynch syndrome) families. *Acta Obstet. Gynecol. Scand.* 90: 437-44.

[85] Renkonen-Sinisalo, L., Butzow, R., Leminen, A., Lehtovirta, P., Mecklin, J. P., Jarvinen, H. J. Surveillance for endometrial cancer in hereditary nonpolyposis colorectal cancer syndrome. *Int. J. Cancer* 12007;120: 821-4.

[86] Vasen, H. F., Blanco, I., Aktan-Collan, K., Gopie, J. P., Alonso, A., Aretz, S., Bernstein, I., Bertario, L., Burn, J., Capella, G., Colas, C., Engel, C., Frayling, I. M., Genuardi, M., Heinimann, K., Hes, F. J., Hodgson, S. V., Karagiannis, J. A., Lalloo, F., Lindblom, A., Mecklin, J. P., Moller, P., Myrhoj, T., Nagengast, F. M., Parc, Y., Ponz de Leon, M., Renkonen-Sinisalo, L., Sampson, J. R., Stormorken, A., Sijmons, R. H., Tejpar, S., Thomas, H. J., Rahner, N., Wijnen, J. T., Jarvinen, H. J., Moslein, G. Revised guidelines for the clinical management of Lynch syndrome (HNPCC): recommendations by a group of European experts. *Gut* 62: 812-23.

[87] Lindor, N. M., Petersen, G. M., Hadley, D. W., Kinney, A. Y., Miesfeldt, S., Lu, K. H., Lynch, P., Burke, W., Press, N. Recommendations for the care of individuals with an inherited predisposition to Lynch syndrome: a systematic review. *JAMA* 12006;296: 1507-17.

[88] Huang, M., Sun, C., Boyd-Rogers, S., Burzawa, J., Milbourne, A., Keeler, E., Yzquierdo, R., Lynch, P., Peterson, S. K., Lu, K. Prospective study of combined colon and endometrial cancer screening in women with lynch syndrome: a patient-centered approach. *J. Oncol. Pract.* 7: 43-7.

[89] Schmeler, K. M., Lynch, H. T., Chen, L. M., Munsell, M. F., Soliman, P. T., Clark, M. B., Daniels, M. S., White, K. G., Boyd-Rogers, S. G., Conrad, P. G., Yang, K. Y., Rubin, M. M., Sun, C. C., Slomovitz, B. M., Gershenson, D. M., Lu, K. H. Prophylactic surgery to reduce the risk of gynecologic cancers in the Lynch syndrome. *N. Engl. J. Med.* 12006;354: 261-9.

[90] Kwon, J. S., Sun, C. C., Peterson, S. K., White, K. G., Daniels, M. S., Boyd-Rogers, S. G., Lu, K. H. Cost-effectiveness analysis of prevention strategies for gynecologic cancers in Lynch syndrome. *Cancer* 12008; 113: 326-35.

[91] Cohen, S. A. Current Lynch Syndrome Tumor Screening Practices: A Survey of Genetic Counselors. *J. Genet. Couns.*

[92] Kwon, J. S., Scott, J. L., Gilks, C. B., Daniels, M. S., Sun, C. C., Lu, K. H. Testing women with endometrial cancer to detect Lynch syndrome. *J. Clin. Oncol.* 29: 2247-52.

In: Endometrial Cancer
Editors: I. Diaz-Padilla, J. Garcia-Donas
ISBN: 978-1-63321-323-4

Chapter III

Endometrial Carcinoma: Pathological and Molecular Features

Xavier Matias-Guiu*

Department of Pathology and Molecular Hospital Universitari Arnau de Vilanova, University of Lleida,
Institute of Biomedical Research in Lleida-IRBLLEIDA

Abstract

There are two main clinico-pathological variants of Endometrial Carcinoma (EC); endometrioid endometrial carcinomas (EEC) (type I), and non-endometrioid endometrial carcinomas (NEEC) (type II). EEC are estrogen-related carcinomas that usually develop in perimenopausal women and coexist or are preceded by complex and atypical endometrial hyperplasia. The vast majority of EEC are low grade tumors (grades 1 and 2), and are associated with good prognosis when they are restricted to the uterus. EEC is the most common type of EC. The microscopical appearance of the tumor resembles that of the proliferative endometrium, with a variable degree of glandular complexity and cellular pleomorphism. Several varieties have been described, including the

* Address for correspondence: Xavier Matias-Guiu, Department of Pathology and Molecular Genetics, Hospital Universitari Arnau de Vilanova, Av Alcalde Rovira Roure 80, 25198 Lleida, Spain

presence of squamous differentiation, villoglandular pattern, secretory features and ciliated cells. Five different molecular features are frequent in this type of tumor, including microsatellite instability, and mutations in PTEN, k-RAS, PIK3CA, FGFR2 and CTNNB1. NEECs are very aggressive, unrelated to estrogen stimulation, arising occasionally in endometrial polyps or from precancerous lesions developing in atrophic endometrium that mainly occur in older women; NEEC include serous (SC) and clear cell carcinoma. NEEC are regarded as high grade tumors, by definition. SC has a high tendency to develop lymph node metastasis and peritoneal spread. In contrast to EEC, NEEC show P53 mutations (90%), inactivation of p16 (40%) and E-cadherin (80-90%), c-erbB2 amplification (30%), alterations in genes involved in the regulation of the mitotic spindle checkpoint (STK15) and loss of heterozygosity at multiple loci, reflecting the presence of chromosomal instability.

Keywords: Endometrial carcinoma, endometrioid, myometrial invasion, molecular features

Endometrial Carcinoma (EC) is heterogeneous. There are different histologic types, with different features at the pathologic and clinical level.

Endometrioid Carcinoma (EEC)

EEC is by far the most common histological type of EC [1, 2]. More than 80% of EC show EEC morphology with variable levels of differentiation and metaplastic changes. EEC is the prototype of Type I EC. Well differentiated (usual-type) EEC is composed of complex glandular structures that resemble to those of the normal proliferative endometrium but are closely packed (back-to-back) [3].

The glands show different shapes ranging from round to oval to angulated and small to large, including cystic change (Figure 1). In high-grade tumors there is a tendency to increase the complexity of the glandular elements that may show fusion and cribriforming or grow in sheets with minimal lumen formation.

A proportion of EECs arise from pre-existing endometrioid hyperplasia [4] However, some cases develop from atrophic [5], or weakly proliferative endometrium. In some other cases, EEC may also arise in a background of a pre-existing endometrial polyp [6].

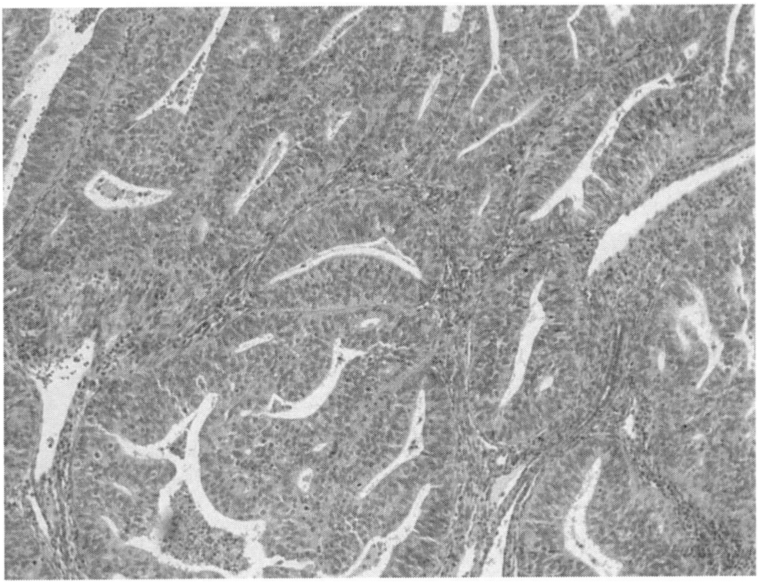

Figure 1. Endometrioid endometrial carcinoma. The tumor glands are irregular and lined by cells with moderate nuclear pleomorphism.

EEC Variants

EEC can show a wide spectrum of morphological features including squamous differentiation, villoglandular arrangement, secretory change and ciliated cells. Almost 50% of EECs show metaplastic changes in the surface, such as microglandular pattern, syncytial aggregates of relatively bland-appearing eosinophilic cells, with papillary or squamous differentiation, or mixed metaplastic changes.

EEC with squamous differentiation accounts for 25-50% of EEC. The presence of squamous differentiation does not affect prognosis. Well-differentiated tumors show intraluminal nests of squamous cells, so-called morules, which can be confluent and may show central necrosis. In contrast, the squamous component of high-grade EECs is characterized by large masses of poorly differentiated tumor cells with few intercellular bridges, well-defined cytoplasmic borders, and prominent eosinophilic or clear cytoplasm. In EECs with squamous differentiation, grading should be done exclusively evaluating the glandular elements. Rarely, they are associated with keratin granulomas in the uterine serosa, adnexa, or peritoneum [8].

Villoglandular EEC accounts for 15-30% of all EECs (2,9,10). They are low grade neoplasms composed of long, slender, delicate papillae with thin fibrovascular cores. The secretory variant, also called, secretory adenocarcinoma, is very uncommon [11]. Tumor cells contain large subnuclear vacuoles.

EEC is the most common EC type in patients with hereditary non-polyposis colon cancer (HNPCC) syndrome (Lynch Syndrome) [12] premenopausal patients being most commonly affected. The HNPCC has its molecular basis in a defect in DNA mismatch repair genes, usually a germline mutation in MLH-1 or MSH-2. Several microscopic features are frequent in EECs in this setting including: 1) poor differentiation, 2) presence of lymphocytes, 3) Crohn-like lymphoid reaction; 4) tendency to lymphovascular invasion, and 5) location in the lower uterine segment. Immunostaining for MLH-1, MSH-2, MSH-6 and PMS-1, as well as microsatellite instability analysis can be helpful to identify the mutated gene. There is some evidence that EEC in the setting of HNPCC syndrome are prone to develop an undifferentiated component, an entity known as dedifferentiated carcinoma (13).

EEC with small non-villous papillae accounts for up to 8% of all EECs (14). It is characterized by the presence of small pseudopapillae lacking fibrovascular cores budding into the lumens of otherwise conventional EEC glands. EEC with microglandular pattern is characterized by a microscopic appearance that simulates microglandular hyperplasia of the cervix (15). Sertoliform EEC is characterized by the presence of a focal or predominant growth of tubules closely mimicking ovarian Sertoli cell tumors (16).

Mucinous Adenocarcinoma

Mucinous carcinoma of the endometrium is very rare and accounts for less than 10% of all EC [17]. As these tumors share similar clinical features with EEC, occurring in women with hyperestrogenism, and a significant proportion of EECs show a variable proportion of mucin-producing cells, mucinous and EECs may represent part of a same spectrum and as such they are frequently linked together. Mucinous carcinoma is characterized by the presence of intracytoplasmatic mucin, in at least 50% of tumor cells.

Serous Carcinoma

Serous carcinoma is a non-endometrioid carcinoma (NEEC), and also the prototype of type II EC. It accounts for 5 – 10% of EC, and presents with stage II or III, often with deep myometrial invasion [18, 19, 20]. The tumor shows thick, fibrotic or edematous papillae with prominent stratification of tumor cells, and cellular budding (Figure 2). The papillae are lined by anaplastic cells with large, eosinophilic cytoplasms. The nuclei are hyperchromatic or vesicular, and contain prominent nucleoli. In some areas, the tumor may show a solid pattern, and in other a glandular arrangement with slit-like and irregular spaces.

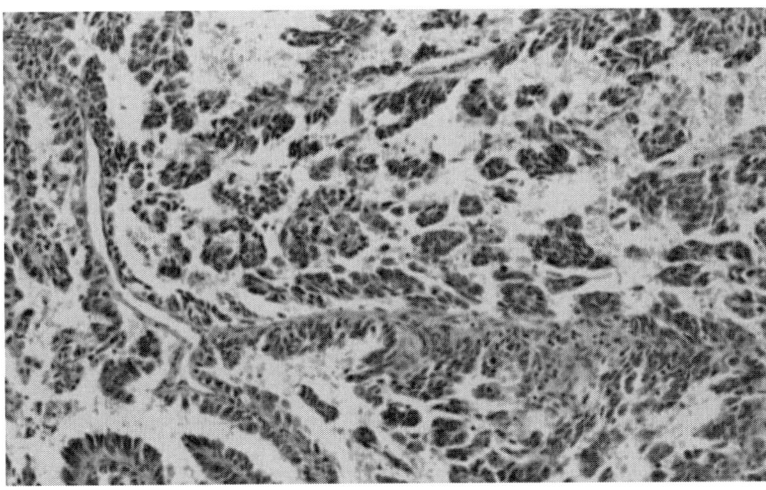

Figure 2. Microscopical apperarance of serous carcinoma.

Psammoma bodies may be present. The tumor is usually associated with deep myometrial invasion, and extensive lymphatic invasion. There is a great tendency to present extrauterine spread at time of diagnosis. Serous carcinoma does not arise from preexisting of endometrial hyperplasia.

The precursor lesion is the so-called Endometrial intraepithelial carcinoma. Both types of lesion usually develop in the setting of atrophic endometrium or endometrial polyps. p53 is one of the molecular abnormalities involved in development and progression of this type of tumors; and tumor cells usually are strongly positive for p53 immunostaining. Ki-67 (MIB-1) is usually strongly positive. WT-1 is usually negative, in contrast with ovarian serous carcinoma.

Clear Cell Carcinoma

Clear cell adenocarcinoma is also a NEEC, prototype of type II EC [21, 22]. Clear cell carcinoma is similar to clear cell carcinomas of the ovary or the cervix. Clear cell adenocarcinoma of the endometrium comprises about 5% of all EC. Microscopically, clear cell adenocarcinomas are characterized by a variety of patterns such as solid, papillary, glandular, and tubulocystic (Figure 3). Most clear cell adenocarcinomas show mixed patterns. Tumor cells may exhibit a prominent clear appearance, with abundant glycogen. Tumor cells may also show a hobnail configuration. Hyaline bodies are very frequent. Clear cell adenocarcinoma usually contains complex papillae with hyalinized cores. The nuclei are pleomorphic, with prominent nucleoli.

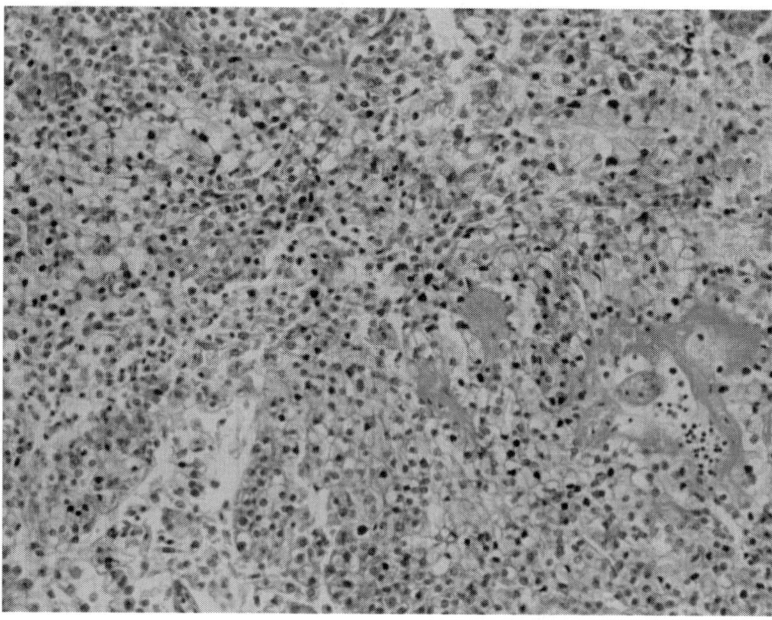

Figure 3. Clear Cell carcinoma.

Mixed Carcinoma

Mixed adenocarcinomas are tumors composed of an admixture of "type I", EECs or their variants (including mucinous carcinoma), and tumor elements of "type II" (serous or clear cell) carcinomas [23]. At least the minor component should comprise 10% of the total volume of the neoplasm. The prognostic significance depends on the proportion of the most aggressive component.

Neuroendocrine Carcinoma

Small cell Neuroendocrine carcinomas are similar to small cell carcinoma of the lung [24]. They contain round or ovoid poorly cohesive cells, with dark clumped chromatin and scanty cytoplasm. The pattern of growth is diffuse, but may exhibit trabeculae, nests or rosette-like structures. There is usually prominent lymphovascular space invasion. They may be positivity for chromogranin A, synaptophysin, CD56, PGP 9.5, vimentin, and cytokeratins. Large cell Neuroendocrine carcinomas are very unusual tumors, similar to large cell carcinoma of the lung [25]. Tumor cells are large, round to polygonal with vesicular or hyperchromatic nuclei with a prominent nucleolus. Tumor cells are arranged in well demarcated nests, trabeculae or cords with peripheral palisading. There are some examples of Combined Neuroendocrine and EC (26), in which large neuroendocrine cells and occasionally small-sized cells, coexist with an EEC or NEEC component.

Undifferentiated Carcinoma

Undifferentiated Carcinoma (UC) of the endometrium was defined as an epithelial tumor that fails to show evidence of either glandular or squamous differentiation. UC represents 1 to 10% of EC [27]. It is characterized by a proliferation of medium-sized, monotonous, epithelial cells growing in solid sheets with no specific pattern. Tumor cells have enlarged nuclei, with prominent nucleoli (Figure 4). Mitosis are frequent. Foci of necrosis are usually present. Tumor cells may show only focal keratin expression, but usually positivity for EMA. The tumor is associated with poor prognosis in the vast majority of the cases. Occasionally, UC arise from pre-existing well- or moderately-differentiated EEC. The term Dedifferentiated Carcinoma (DDC) has been used to designate such special type of tumor [28].

Molecular Features of EC

It has been demonstrated that the molecular genetic alterations involved in the development of EEC (type I) differ from those of NEEC (type II) [29-32] (Table I). Whereas EEC shows microsatellite instability (MI) and mutations in the PTEN, PIK3CA, K-RAS, and beta-catenin genes, NEEC have alterations of p53, loss of heterozygosity (LOH) on several chromosomes, as well as other molecular alterations (STK15, p16, E-cadherin, and C-erbB2)

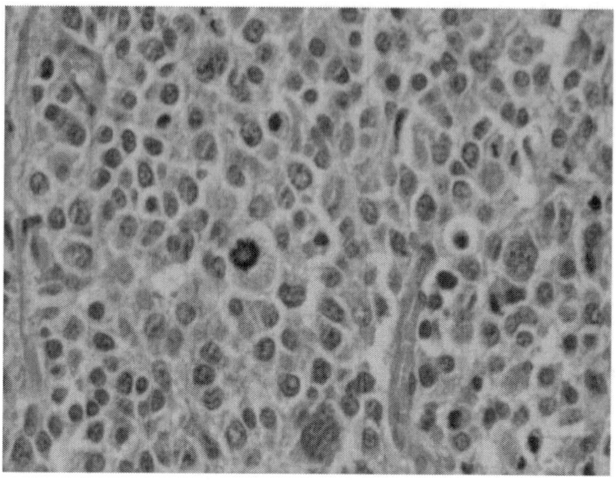

Figure 4. Undifferentiated carcinoma. Notice presence of highly atypical cells.

Microsatellite instability (MI) was initially noted in cancers of patients with the hereditary non-polyposis colorectal carcinoma (HNPCC), but also in sporadic colon cancers. EC is the second most common tumor found in HNPCC patients. MI is seen in 75% of EC associated with HNPCC, but also in 25-30% of sporadic EC (33-36). HNPCC patients have an inherited germline mutation in MLH1, MSH2, MSH6 or PMS2. MI occurs more frequently in EEC (30%) than in NEEC. In sporadic tumors, MLH1 inactivation by promoter hypermethylation is the main cause of mismatch repair deficiency [37]. The MI-associated mismatch repair deficiency leads to the accumulation of mutations in coding and non-coding DNA sequences. Some small short-tandem repeats, like mononucleotide repeats, located within the coding sequence of some important genes; (BAX, IGFIIR, MSH3, MSH6, MBD4, CHK1, CASP5,) are targets in the process of tumor progression of MI+ EC. Mutations in these tracts are interpreted as secondary events in cancers with MI [38, 39].

Table 1. Molecular alterations in type I EC and type II EC

Biomarker	Alteration	Frequency in Type I EC %	Frequency in type II EC %
PTEN	Loss of function	40-80	0-10
KRAS	mutation	10-25	2-4
KRAS	amplification	2	10
CTNNB4/ β-catenin	Mutation/nuclear expression	20-50	0-5
MI	Microsatellite Instability	20-45	0-5
FGFR-2	Mutation	10-16	1
PIK3CA	Mutation	30	20
PIK3CA	Amplification	2-14	46
ER, PR	Expression	70-73	20-24
PIK3RI	mutation	20	0
PIK3R2	mutation	5	25
AKT	mutation	3	0
ARID1A	Mutation/loss of function	19	6
EGFR	overexpression	46	34
Stathmin	overexpression	15	64
HER 2	overexpression	3-10	32
E-cadherin	Loss of function	5-50	60-90
P16	Loss of function	8	45
PPP2R1A	mutation	5	15-40
Cyclin D1/E	amplification	2-5	26-42
P53	mutation	10-20	80-90

The tumor suppressor gene PTEN is frequently abnormal in EC [40-41]. LOH at chromosome 10q23 occurs in 40% of EC [42]. Somatic PTEN mutations are also common in EC, and they are almost exclusively restricted to EEC, occurring in 37-61% of them and lead to activation of the PI3K/AKT pathway. There are many evidences showing that EECs with mutations in PTEN have genomic instability [43]. For that reason, some authors have suggested to treat patients with PARP inhibitors [44]. Mutations in PIK3CA may contribute to the alteration of the PI3K/AKT signalling pathway in EC [45-47]. PI3K is a heterodimeric enzyme consisting of a catalytic subunit (p110) and a regulatory subunit (p85). The PIK3CA gene codes for the p110 catalytic subunit of PI3K. A high frequency of mutations in the PIK3CA gene has been reported recently in EC. Mutations are predominantly located in the helical (exon 9) and kinase (exon 20) domains, but they can occur also in exons 1 to 7 [48]. PIK3CA mutations occur in 24-39% of the cases, and coexisted frequently with PTEN mutations. PIK3CA mutations, particularly in exon 20, have been associated with adverse prognostic factors such as high-grade and myometrial invasion. Although initially described in EEC, PI3KCA mutations also occur in NEEC, and also mixed EEC-NEEC [49-50]. Furthermore, gene expression profile differences in the PI3K-AKT signalling pathway identify two subgroups of high-grade EC with different molecular alterations (PI3K/AKT pathway versus p53 alterations) which may play distinct roles in endometrial carcinogenesis [51]. Moreover, mutations in PIK3RI (p85α), the inhibitory subunit of PI3K, have been detected in 43% of EEC, and 12% of NEEC [52].

Among AKT targets, downstream effector mTOR is of particular interest. mTOR inhibitors have been recently developed as potential anticancer agents. Tumors associated with PTEN inactivation, like EC, are particularly susceptible to the therapeutic effects of mTOR inhibitors. Pharmacological inhibition of mTOR in PTEN+/- mice has shown reduced neoplastic proliferation, tumor size, and S6K activity [53]. Moreover, the use of dual PI3K-mTOR has been proposed as a targeted therapy, since they may target p110α, β, and δ isoforms, mTORC1 and mTORC2 [54].

The RAS-RAF-MEK-ERK signaling pathway plays an important role in EC. The frequency of K-RAS mutations in EC ranges between 10 to 30% [55]. BRAF, another member of the RAS-RAF-MEK-ERK pathways is very infrequently mutated in EC [56]. Recent studies have demonstrated that RASSF1A inactivation by promoter hypermethylation may contribute significantly to increased activity of the RAS-RAF-MEK-ERK signaling pathway [57].

There are several evidences suggesting that the FGF signaling pathway is important in EC. Recent studies have shown that EC presents frequent inactivation of SPRY-2, a protein that is involved in the negative regulation of the FGFR pathway [58]. Moreover, somatic mutations in FGFR2 have been recently detected in 10-12% of EC, particularly in EEC (16%) [59-61].

Mutations in exon 3 of beta-catenin gene (CTNNB1) occur in 14% to 44% of EC [62-64], and result in stabilization of the protein, cytoplasmic and nuclear accumulation, and participation in signal transduction and transcriptional activation through the formation of complexes with DNA binding proteins. Mutations are homogeneously distributed in different areas of the tumors, which suggest that they do play a role in early steps of endometrial tumorigenesis. The presence of a cytoplasmic and nuclear beta-catenin immunoreactivity in some ECs that did not show a mutation in

CTNNB1 suggests that alterations in other genes of the Wnt/beta-catenin/LEF-1 pathway may be responsible for the stabilization and putative transcription activator role of beta-catenin in these tumors [65, 66].

In contrast to EEC, NEEC show P53 mutations (90%), inactivation of p16 (40%) and E-cadherin (80-90%), c-erbB2 amplification (30%), alterations in genes involved in the regulation of the mitotic spindle checkpoint (STK15) and loss of heterozygosity at multiple loci, reflecting the presence of chromosomal instability [67-71]. While P53 mutations occur in 90% of NEEC, they are only present in 10-20% of EEC, which are mostly grade 3 tumors. Inactivation of the cell cycle regulator p16 is also more frequent in NEEC (40%) than in EEC (10%). The underlying mechanism is not clear, but probably involves deletion and promoter hypermethylation. Reduced expression of E-cadherin is frequent in EC, and may be caused by LOH or promoter hypermethylation. In fact, LOH at 16q22.1 is seen in almost 60% of NEEC, but only in 22% of EEC. C-erbB2 overexpression and amplification are also seen more frequently in NEEC (43% and 29%) than in EEC. However, the most typical molecular feature of NEEC is chromosomal instability. This phenomenon is characterized by the presence of widespread chromosomal gains and losses, which reflect the presence of aneuploidy. cDNA arrays have demonstrated that NEEC usually show up-regulation of genes (STK15, BUB1, CCNB2) that are involved in the regulation of the mitotic spindle checkpoint.

Among NEEC, clear cell carcinomas show specific features. Based on the similarities between ovarian and endometrial clear cell carcinoma, it has been suggested that both types of tumors may exhibit similar alterations, including mutations in PIK3CA and PTEN. Mutation of the ARID1A gene and loss of the corresponding protein BAF250a has recently been described as a frequent event in clear cell and EECs of the ovary. In a recent study, these changes have been found in 29% of grade 1 or 2 and 39% of grade 3 EEC, 18% of uterine serous carcinomas and 26% of uterine clear cell carcinomas. In a different study, uterine low-grade EEC have also shown a relatively high-frequency loss of ARID1A expression (26%) and ARID1A mutations (40%) [72, 73].

cDNA array studies have demonstrated that the expression profiling of EEC is different from that of NEEC [74-79]. In one study, 191 genes exhibited a >2-fold differences between 10 EECs and 16 NEECs. One of the genes, TFF3 was significantly up-regulated in EECs, while increased expression of FOLR was seen in NEECs. In a different study, a different expression profile was seen between EEC and NEEC, and the differences involved 66 genes.

Interestingly, estrogen-regulated genes were up-regulated in EEC, whereas NEEC showed increased expression of genes involved in the regulation of the mitotic spindle checkpoint. A third study demonstrated differentially expression of 1,055 genes between EECs and serous carcinomas. Genes up-regulated in serous carcinomas were IGF2, PTGS1 and p16, while genes up-regulated in EEC included TFF3, FOXA2, and MSX2. A different study identified 315 genes that statistically differentiated EEC from NEEC. Moreover, a different expression profile was also found between EC associated with microsatellite instability and stable EC. Interestingly, two members of the secreted frizzled related protein family (SFRP1 and SFRP4) were more frequently down-regulated in EC with microsatellite instability. In a different study, it was seen that the tumors (ovarian and uterine) with beta-catenin alterations, showed common gene expression profile. Our group has also identified, by c-DNA array studies, up-regulation of RUNX1/AML1 and ERM/ETV5 in EC [80], and suggested an implication of such genes in myometrial invasion. One study compared the expression profiles of similar histological subtypes of ovarian and endometrial carcinomas; and showed that clear cell carcinomas had a very similar profile, regardless of the organ of origin. In contrast, differences were seen when comparing endometrioid and serous carcinomas of ovarian and endometrial origin.

The Cancer Genome Atlas Research Network (TCGA) has recently performed an integrating genomic characterization of EC, after having evaluated a series of 373 tumors by different methods, including copy number analysis, DNA (exome and genome) sequencing, RNA sequencing, reverse phase protein assays, miRNA sequencing, and DNA methylation analysis [81]. Results of this study show that unsupervised hierarchical clustering of somatic copy number alterations grouped the tumors in four clusters. Cluster I tumors were nearly devoid of copy number alterations and was composed of EEC. Clusters 2 and 3 were also composed of EEC, but exhibited specific alterations (amplification of IGF1R in cluster 2, and amplification of 1q in cluster 3). Cluster 4 was composed of the majority of serous and mixed carcinomas, but also 12% of EEC (particularly, grade 3EEC), and exhibited high degree of gene copy number alterations. More interestingly, exome sequence analysis revealed four groups of tumors. Group 1, with EEC with mutations in POLE, and showing high mutation rates (ultramutated), associated with good prognosis. Group 2, including EEC with microsatellite instability (hypermutated), and group 3 tumors including EEC with low copy number alterations, showing similar progression-free survival rates. Group 4 (Serous-like) including serous carcinomas, but also some EEC (usually grade 3), exhibiting p53 mutations, and worse prognosis. Results show that there is a group of EEC, which are molecularly and prognostically similar to serous carcinoma.

Molecular Features of EC Not Fitting within the Dualistic (Type I Versus Type II) Model

The classification of EC into two groups (type I and type II) is artificial and too rigid and the dualistic model has been recently challenged (Figure 5). In daily practice, pathologists are faced with tumors showing combined or hybrid morphologic and molecular characteristics. Furthermore, even if serous and clear cell carcinomas have been classify within the same category of tumors as they are more aggressive than EC, recent studies have shown that these are in fact distinct tumor types, as they exhibit different clinical, immunohistochemical and molecular features. When an EC has an admixture of EEC and EC, with the minor component representing at least 10% of the neoplasm, the tumor should be classified as a mixed carcinoma.

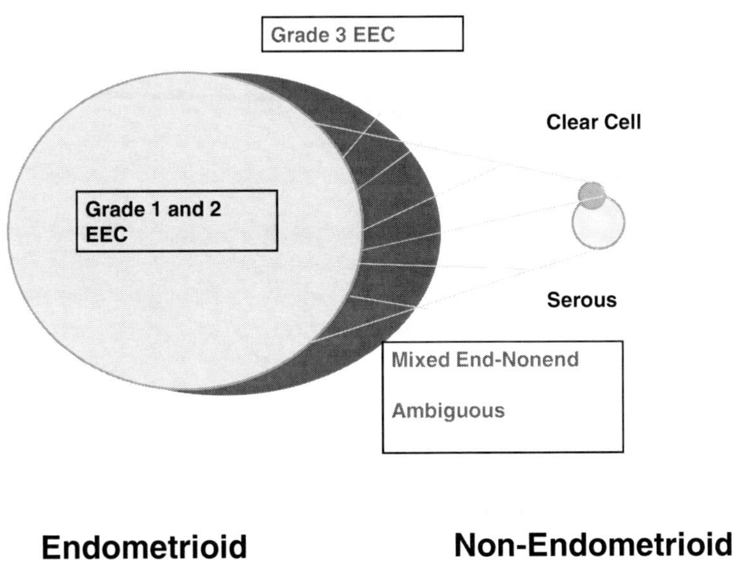

Figure 5. There is overlapping at the morphologic and molecular levels between EEC and NEEC.

Based on molecular analysis, it has been suggested that the NEEC component originates as a result of tumor progression from a pre-existing EEC, since frequently these tumors retain the molecular alterations of typical EEC. There are some tumors that exhibit overlapping and intermediate features between EEC and NEEC and fail to show two distinct components. The term "EC with ambiguous features" has been proposed for these carcinomas [82]. Their clinical and molecular features should be defined better.

Occasionally, undifferentiated carcinomas arise from pre-existing well- or moderately-differentiated EEC. The term Dedifferentiated Carcinoma (DDC) has been used to designate such special type of tumor. Several groups of investigators have reported that the EECs with a tendency to develop a high-grade, undifferentiated carcinoma present microsatellite instability as a frequent molecular genetic alteration [83].

Malignant Mixed Müllerian Tumors (MMMT), (carcinosarcoma), are uncommon uterine neoplasms. They are composed by a bifasic pattern, with epithelial malignant elements and a sarcomatoid component (Figure 6).

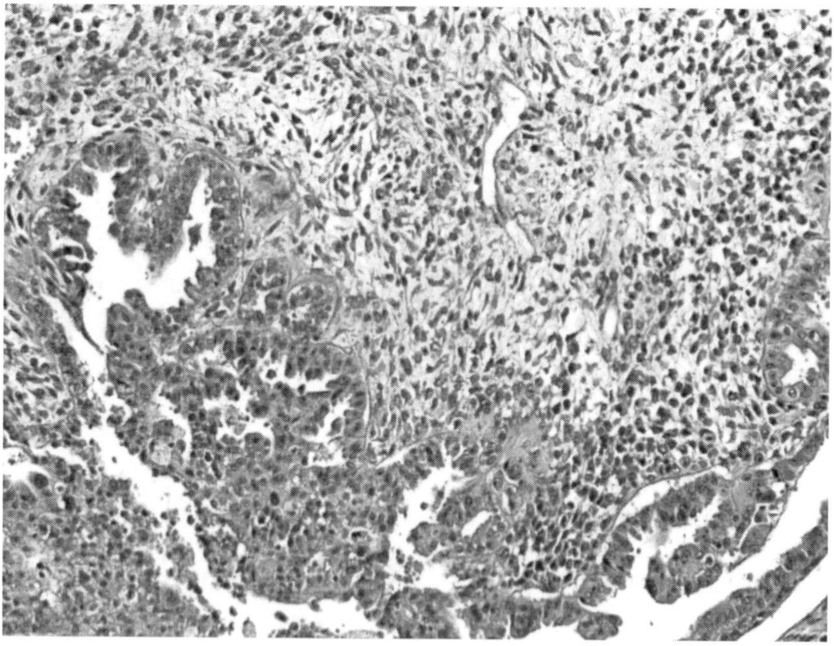

Figure 6. Malignant Mixed Müllerian Tumor.

It has recently suggested from the molecular point of view that MMMT should be regarded as metaplastic carcinomas. Like sarcomatoid carcinomas of other locations, carcinosarcomas probably develop through epithelial-to-mesenchymal transition (EMT) in EC. Whereas the transient occurrence of the EMT phenomenon is important for myometrial invasion in conventional EC, MMMT show permanent expression of EMT leading to repression of epithelial markers (E-cadherin) and increased expression of mesenchymal markers including proteins involved in skeletal muscle development. All of these molecular changes are responsible for the appearance of the sarcomatous areas as well as the presence of heterologous differentiation. It has been recently seen that MMMT show HMGA2 overexpression, and a microRNA signature typical of EMT [84, 85].

References

[1] Bockman JV: Two pathogenetic types of endometrial carcinoma. *Gynecol. Oncol.* 1983; 15:10-7.

[2] Tavasoli FA, Devilee P: Pathology and Genetics of Tumours of the breast and female organs. WHO classification of tumours. *IARC press*, Lyon 2003.

[3] Clement PhB, Young RH, EEC of the uterus: A review of its pathology with emphasis on recent advances and problematic aspects. *Adv. Anat. Pathol.* 2002 3:145-84.

[4] Sherman ME, Silverberg SG. Advances in endometrial pathology. *Clin. Lab. Med.* 1995 15:517-43.

[5] Sivridis E, Giatromanolaki A. The endometrial hyperplasias revisited. *Virchows Arch.* 2008 453:223-31.

[6] Salm R The incidence and significance of early carcinomas in endometrial polyps. *J. Pathol.* 1972 108:47-53.

[7] Jacques SM, Qureshi F, Lawrence WD, Surface epithelial changes in endometrial adenocarcinoma: diagnostic pitfalls in curettage specimens. Int J Gynecol Pathol. 1995 14:191-78. Kim KR, Scully RE. Peritoneal keratin granulomas with carcinomas of endometrium and ovary and atypical polypoid adenomyoma of endometrium. A clinicopathologycal analysis od 22 cases. *Am. J. Surg. Pathol.* 1990;14:925-32.

[8] Ambros RA, Malfetano JH. Villoglandular adenocarcinoma of the endometrium. *Am. J. Surg. Pathol.* 1998;22:1379-85.

[9] Ambros RA, Ballouk F, Malfetano JH, et al. Significance of papillary (villoglandular) differentiation in EEC of the uterus. *Am. J. Surg. Pathol.* 1994;18:569-75.

[10] Tobon H, Watkins GJ. Secretory adenocarcinoma of the endometrium. *Int. J. Gynecol. Pathol.* 1985;4:328-35.

[11] Garg K and Soslow RA. Lynch Syndrome (hereditary non-polyposis colorectal cancer) and endometrial carcinoma. *J. Clin. Pathol.* 2009;62:679-84.

[12] Tafe LJ, Garg K, Chew I, Tornos C, Soslow RA. Endometrial and ovarian carcinomas with undifferentiated components: clinically aggressive and frequently underrecognized neoplasms. *Mod. Pathol.* 2010;23:781-9.

[13] Murray SK, Young RH, Scully RE. Uterine EEC with small nonvillous papillae: an analysis of 26 cases of a favourable-prognosis tumor to be distinguished from serous carcinoma. *Int. J. Surg. Pathol.* 2000;8:279-89.

[14] Young RH, Scully RE. Uterine carcinomas simulating microglandular hyperplasia: a report of six cases. *Am. J. Surg. Pathol.* 1992;16:1092-7.

[15] Eichlom JH, Young RH, Clement PB. Sertoliform endometrial adenocarcinoma: a study of four cases. *Int. J. Gynecol. Pathol.* 1996;15:119-26.

[16] Melhem MF, Tobon H. Mucinous adenocarcinoma of the endometrium: a clinicopathologycal review of 8 cases. *Int. J. Gynecol. Pathol.* 1987;6:347-55.

[17] Clement PB, Young RH. Non-endometrioid carcinomas of the uterine corpus: a review of their pathology with emphasis on recent advances and problematic aspects. *Adv. Anat. Pathol.* 2004;11:117-142.

[18] Sherman ME, Bitterman P, Rosenshein NB, Delgado G, Kurman RJ. Uterine serous carcinoma. A morphologically diverse neoplasm with unifying clinicopathologic features. *Am. J. Surg. Pathol.* 1992;16:600-610.

[19] Prat J, Oliva E, Lerma E, Vaquero M, Matias-Guiu X. Uterine papillary serous adenocarcinoma. A 10-case study of p53 and c-erbB-2 expression and DNA content. *Cancer.* 1994;74:1778-1783.

[20] Kanbour-Shakir A, Tobon H. Primary clear cell carcinoma of the endometrium: a clinicopathologic study of 20 cases. *Int. J. Gynecol.* Pathol. 1991;10:67-78.

[21] Abeler VM, Vergote IB, Kjorstad KE, Trope CG. Clear cell carcinoma of the endometrium. Prognosis and metastatic pattern. *Cancer.* 1996;78:1740-1747.

[22] Quddus MR, Sung CJ, Zhang C, et al.: Minor serous and clear cell components adversely affect prognosis in "mixed-type" endometrial carcinomas: a clinicopathologic study of 36 stage-I cases. *Reprod. Sci.* 17:673-678, 2010.

[23] Van Hoeven KH, Hudock JA, Woodruff JM, Suhrland M. Small cell neuroendocrine carcinoma of the endometrium. *Int. J. Gynecol. Pathol.* 1995;14;21-29.

[24] Deodhar KK, Kerkar RA, Suryawanshi P, Menon H, Menon S. Large cell neuroendocrine carcinoma of the endometrium: an extremely uncommon diagnosis, but worth the efforts. *J. Cancer Res. Ther.* 2011 7:211-3.

[25] Mulvanny NJ, Allen DG. Combined large cell neuroendocrine and endometrioid carcinoma of the endometrium. *Int. J. Gynecol. Pathol.* 2008;27;49-.

[26] Abeler VM, Kjorstad KE, Nesland JM. Undifferentiated carcinoma of the endometrium. A histopathologic and clinical study of 31 cases. *Cancer.* 1991;68:98-105.

[27] Silva EG, Deavers MT, Bodurka DC, Malpica A: Association of low-grade endometrioid carcinoma of the uterus and ovary with undifferentiated carcinoma: a new type of dedifferentiated carcinoma?. *Int. J. Gynecol. Pathol.* 2005 25:52-58.

[28] Bokhman JV. Two pathogenetic types of endometrial carcinoma. *Gynecol. Oncol.* 1983; 15:10-17.

[29] Matias-Guiu X, Catasús L, Bussaglia E, Lagarda H, Garcia A, Pons C, Muñoz J, Garcia A, Pons C, Muñoz J, Argüelles R, Machin P, Prat J. Molecular Pathology of endometrial hyperplasia and carcinoma. *Hum. Pathol.* 2001; 32:569-77.

[30] Prat J, Gallardo A, Cuatrecasas M, Catasús L. Endometrial carcinoma: pathology and genetics. *Pathology.* 2007; 39:72-87.

[31] Llobet D, Pallares J, Yeramian A, Santacana M, Eritja N, Velasco A, Dolcet X, Matias-Guiu X. Molecular pathology of endometrial carcinoma; practical aspects from the diagnostic and therapeutical view points. *J. Clin. Pathol.* 2009; 62:777-85.

[32] Duggan BD, Felix JC, Muderspach LI, Tourgeman D, Zheng J, Shibata D. Microsatellite instability in sporadic endometrial carcinoma. *J. Natl. Cancer Inst.* 1994; 86:1216-21.

[33] Kobayashi K, Sagae S, Kudo H, Koi S, Nakamura Y. Microsatellite instability in endometrial carcinomas: frequent replication errors in tumors of early onset and/or of poorly differentiated type. *Genes. Chromosom. Cancer 1995*; 14:128-32.

[34] Risinger JI, Berchuck A, Kohler MF, Watson P, Lynch HT, Boyd J. Genetic instability of microsatellites in endometrial carcinoma. *Cancer Res.* 1993; 53:5100-3.

[35] Catasús L, Machin P, Matias-Guiu X, Prat J. Microsatellite instability in endometrial carcinomas clinicopathologic correlations in a series of 42 cases. *Human Pathol.* 1998; 29:1160-4.

[36] Esteller M, Catasús Ll, Matias-Guiu X, Mutter GL, Prat J, Baylin SB, Herman JG. hMLH1 promoter hypermethylation is an early event in human endometrial tumorigenesis. *Am. J. Pathol.* 1999; 155:1767-72.

[37] Catasús L, Matias-Guiu X, Machin P, Muñoz J, Prat J. BAX somatic framshift mutations in endometrioid adenocarcinomas of the endometrium: evidence for a tumor progression role in endometrioid carcinomas with microsatellite instability. *Lab. Invest.* 1998; 78:1439-44.

[38] Catasús L, Matias-Guiu X, Machin P, Zannoni GF, Scambia G, Benedetti Panici PL, Prat J: Frameshift mutations at coding mononucleotide repeat microsatellites in endometrial carcinomas with microsatellite instability. *Cancer* 2000; 88:2290-7.

[39] Mutter GL, Lin MC, Fitzgerald JT, Kum JB, Baak JPA Lees, Weng LP, Eng Ch. Altered PTEN expression as a Diagnostic Marker for the Earliest Endometrial Precancers. *J. Natl. Cancer Inst.* 2000; 92:924-31

[40] Bussaglia E, del Rio E, Matias-Guiu X, Prat J. PTEN mutations in endometrial carcinomas. A molecular and clinicopathologic analysis of 38 cases. *Hum. Pathol.* 2000; 31:312-7.

[41] Nagase S, Sato S, Tezuka F, Wada Y, Yajima A, Horii A. Deletion mapping on chromosome 10q25-q26 in human endometrial cancer. *Br. J. Cance*r 1996; 74:1979-83.

[42] Shen WH, Balajee AS, Wang J, Wu H, Eng C, Pandolfi PP, Yin Y. Essential role for nuclear PTEN in maintaining chromosomal integrity. *Cell.* 2007 ;128:157-70.

[43] Dedes KJ, Wetterskog D, Mendes-Pereira AM, Natrajan R, Lambros MB, Geyer FC, Vatcheva R, Savage K, Mackay A, Lord CJ, Ashworth A, Reis-Filho JS. PTEN deficiency in endometrioid endometrial adenocarcinomas predicts sensitivity to PARP inhibitors. *Sci. Transl. Med.* 2010 2:53ra75.

[44] Oda K, Stokoe D, Taketani Y, McCormick F. High frequency of coexistent mutations of PIK3CA and PTEN genes in endometrial carcinoma. *Cancer Res.* 2005; 65:10669-73.

[45] Velasco A, Bussaglia E, Pallares J, Dolcet X, Llobet D, Encinas M, Llecha N, Palacios J, Prat J, Matias-Guiu X. PIK3CA gene mutations in endometrial carcinoma: correlation with PTEN and K-RAS alterations. *Hum Pathol.* 2006; 37:1465-72.

[46] Catasús L, Gallardo A, Cuatrecasas M, Prat J. PIK3CA mutations in the kinase domain (exon 20) of uterine endometrial adenocarcinomas are associated with adverse prognostic parameters. *Mod. Pathol.* 2008; 21:131-9.

[47] Rudd ML, Price JC, Fogoros S, Godwin AK, Sgroi DC, Merino MJ, Bell DW. A unique spectrum of somatic PIK3CA (p110alpha) mutations within primary endometrial carcinomas. *Clin. Cancer Res.* 2011; 17:1331-40.

[48] Catasús L, Gallardo A, Cuatrecasas M, Prat J. Concomitant PI3K-AKT and p53 alterations in endometrial carcinomas are associated with poor prognosis. *Mod. Pathol.* 2009; 22:522-9.

[49] Hayes MP, Douglas W, Ellenson LH. Molecular alterations of EGFR and PIK3CA in uterine serous carcinoma. *Gynecol. Oncol.* 2009; 113:370-3.

[50] Catasús L, D'Angelo E, Pons C, Espinosa I, Prat J. Expression profiling of 22 genes involved in the PI3K-AKT pathway identifies two subgroups of high-grade endometrial carcinomas with different molecular alterations. *Mod. Pathol.* 2010 23:694-702.

[51] Urick ME, Rudd ML, Godwin AK, Sgroi D, Merino M, Bell DW PIK3R1 (p85α) is somatically mutated at high frequency in primary endometrial cancer. *Cancer Res.* 2011 15;71:4061-7.

[52] Milam MR, Celestino J, Wu W, Broaddus RR, Schmeler KM, Slomovitz BM, Soliman PT, Gershenson DM, Wang H, Ellenson LH, Lu KH. Reduced progression of endometrial hyperplasia with oral mTOR inhibition in the Pten heterozygote murine model. *Am. J. Obstet. Gynecol.* 2007; 196:247.e1-5.

[53] Serra V, Markman B, Scaltriti M, Eichhorn PJ, Valero V, Guzman M, Botero ML, Llonch E, Atzori F, Di Cosimo S, Maira M, Garcia-Echeverria C, Parra JL, Arribas J, Baselga J. NVP-BEZ235, a dual PI3K/mTOR inhibitor, prevents PI3K signaling and inhibits the growth of cancer cells with activating PI3K mutations. *Cancer Res.* 2008 68:8022-30.

[54] Lagarda H, Catasús L, Argüelles R, Matias-Guiu X, Prat, J. K-ras mutations in endometrial carcinoma with microsatellite instabilit. *J. Pathol.* 2001; 193:193-9.

[55] Moreno-Bueno G, Sanchez-Estevez C, Palacios J, Hardisson D, Shiozawa T.Low frequency of BRAF mutations in endometrial and in cervical carcinomas. *Clin. Cancer Res.* 2006; 15;12:3865.

[56] Pallarés J, Velasco A, Eritja N, Santacana M, Dolcet X, Cuatrecasas M, Palomar-Asenjo V, Catasús L, Prat J, Matias-Guiu X.Promoter hypermethylation and reduced expression of RASSF1A are frequent molecular alterations of endometrial carcinoma. *Mod. Pathol.* 2008; 21:691-9.

[57] Velasco A, Pallares J, Santacana M, Gatius S, Fernandez M, Domingo M, Valls J, Yeramian A, Encinas M, Dolcet X, Matias-Guiu X. Promoter hypermethylation and expression of sprouty 2 in endometrial carcinoma. *Hum. Pathol.* 2011; 42:185-93.

[58] Pollock PM, Gartside MG, Dejeza LC, Powell MA, Mallon MA, Mohammadi M, Futreal PA, Stratton MR, Trent JM, Goodfelow PJ. Frequent activating FGFR2 mutations in endometrial carcinomas parallel germline mutations associated with craniosynostosis and skeletal dysplasia syndromes. *Oncogene* 2007; 26:7158-62.

[59] Dutt A, Salvesen HB, Chen TH, Ramos AH, Onofrio RC, Hatton C, Nicoletti R, Winckler W, Grewal R, Hanna M, Wyhs N, Ziaugra L, Richter DJ, Trovik J, Engelsen IB, Stefansson IM, Fennell T, Cibulskis K, Zody MC, Akslen LA, Gabriel S, Wong KK, Sellers WR, Meyerson M, Greulich H. Drug-sensitive FGFR2 mutations in endometrial carcinoma. *Proc. Natl. Acad. Sci. U S A.* 2008; 105:8713-7.

[60] Gatius S, Velasco A, Azueta A, Santacana M, Pallares J, Valls J, Dolcet X, Prat J, Matias-Guiu X. FGFR-2 alterations in endometrial carcinoma. *Mod. Pathol.* 2011; 24:1500-10.

[61] Fukuchi T, Sakamoto M, Tsuda H, Maruyama K, Nozawa S, Hirohashi S. Beta-catenin mutations in carcinoma of the uterine endometrium. *Cancer Res.* 1998; 58:3526-8.

[62] Kobayashi K, Sagae S, Nishioka Y, Tokino T, Kudo R. Mutations of the beta-catenin gene in endometrial carcinomas. *Jpn. J. Cancer Res.* 1999; 90:55-9.

[63] Machin P, Catasús L, Pons C, Muñoz J, Matias-Guiu X, Prat J. CTNNB1 mutations and beta-catenin expression in endometrial carcinomas. *Human Pathol.* 2002; 33:206-12.

[64] Palacios J, Moreno-Bueno G, Catasús L, Matias-Guiu X, Prat J, Gamallo C. Beta and gamma-catenin expression in endometrial carcinoma. Relationship with clinicopathological features and microsatellite instability. *Virchows Arch.* 2001; 193:193-9.

[65] Moreno-Bueno G, Hardisson D, Sánchez C, Sarrió D, Cassia R, García-Rostán G, Prat J, Guo M, Herman JG, Matías-Guiu X, Esteller M, Palacios J. Abnormalities of the APC/beta-catenin pathway in endometrial cancer. *Oncogene.* 2002; 14; 21:7981-90.

[66] Tashiro H, Isacson C, Levine R, Kurman RJ, Cho KR, Hedrick L. P53 gene mutations are common in uterine serous carcinoma and occurs early in their pathogenesis. *Am. J. Pathol* 1997; 150:177-85.

[67] Sherman ME, Bur ME, Kurman RJ. P53 in endometrial cancer and its putative precursors: Evidence for diverse pathways of tumorigenesis. *Human Pathol.* 1995; 26:1268-74.

[68] Hayes MP, Ellenson LH. Molecular alterations in uterine serous carcinoma. *Gynecol. Oncol.* 2010; 116:286-9.

[69] Morrison C, Zanagnolo V, Ramirez N, Cohn DE, Kelbick N, Copeland L, Maxwell GL, Fowler JM. HER-2 is an independent prognostic factor in endometrial cancer: association with outcome in a large cohort of surgically staged patients. *J. Clin. Oncol.* 2006; 24:2376-85.

[70] Tritz D, Pieretti M, Turner S, Powell D. Loss of heterozygosity in usual and special variant carcinomas of the endometrium. *Hum. Pathol.* 1997, 28:607-12.

[71] Guan B, Mao TL, Panuganti PK, Kuhn E, Kurman RJ, Maeda D, Chen E, Jeng YM, Wang TL, Shih IeM. Mutation and Loss of Expression of ARID1A in Uterine Low-grade Endometrioid Carcinoma. *Am. J. Surg. Pathol.* 2011; 35:625-32.

[72] Wiegand KC, Lee AF, Al-Agha OM, Chow C, Kalloger SE, Scott DW, Steidl C, Wiseman SM, Gascoyne RD, Gilks B, Huntsman DG. Loss of BAF250a (ARID1A) is frequent in high-grade endometrial carcinomas. *J. Pathol.* 2011; 224:328-33.

[73] Risinger JI, Maxwell GL, Chandramouli GV, Jazaeri A, Aprelikova O, Patterson T, Berchuck A, Barrett JC. Microarray analysis reveals distinct gene expression profiles among different histologic types of endometrial cancer. *Cancer Res.* 2003; 63:6-11.

[74] Bignotti E, Ravaggi A, Tassi RA, Calza S, Rossi E, Falchetti M, Romani C, Bandiera E, Odicino FE, Pecorelli S, Santin AD. Trefoil factor 3: a novel serum marker identified by gene expression profiling in high-grade endometrial carcinomas. *Brit. J. Cancer* 2008 99, 768–773.

[75] Dainty LA, Risinger JI, Morrison C, Chandramouli GV, Bidus MA, Zahn C, Rose GS, Fowler J, Berchuck A, Maxwell GL Overexpression of folate binding protein and mesothelin are associated with uterine serous carcinoma. *Gynecol. Oncol.* 2007 105:563-7

[76] Moreno-Bueno G, Sánchez-Estévez C, Cassia R, Rodríguez-Perales S, Díaz-Uriarte R, Domínguez O, Hardisson D, Andujar M, Prat J, Matias-Guiu X, Cigudosa JC, Palacios J. Differential gene expression profile in endometrioid and nonendometrioid endometrial carcinoma: STK15 is frequently overexpressed and amplified in nonendometrioid carcinomas.*Cancer Res.* 2003; 63:5697-702.

[77] Risinger JI, Maxwell GL, Chandramouli GV, Aprelikova O, Litzi T, Umar A, Berchuck A, Barrett JC. Gene expression profiling of microsatellite unstable and microsatellite stable endometrial cancers indicates distinct pathways of aberrant signaling. *Cancer Res.* 2005; 65:5031-7.

[78] Yao Y, Chen Y, Wang Y, Li X, Wang J, Shen D, Wei L. Molecular classification of human endometrial cancer based on gene expression profiles from specialized microarrays. *Int. J. Gynaecol. Obstet.* 2010 110:125-9.

[79] Planagumà J, Díaz-Fuertes M, Gil-Moreno A, Abal M, Monge M, García A, Baró T, Thomson TM, Xercavins J, Alameda F, Reventós J. A differential gene expression profile reveals overexpression of RUNX1/AML1 in invasive endometrioid carcinoma. *Cancer Res.* 2004; 64:8846-53.

[80] Cancer Genome Atlas Research Network, Kandoth C, Schultz N, Cherniack AD, Akbani R, Liu Y, Shen H, Robertson AG, Pashtan I, Shen R, Benz CC, Yau C, Laird PW, Ding L, Zhang W, Mills GB, Kucherlapati R, Mardis ER, Levine DA. Integrated genomic characterization of endometrial carcinoma. *Nature.* 2013 497:67-73.

[81] Soslow RA Endometrial carcinomas with ambiguous features. Semin *Diagn. Pathol.* 2010; 27:261-73.

[82] Tafe LJ, Garg K, Chew I, Tornos C, Soslow RA. Endometrial and ovarian carcinomas with undifferentiated components: clinically aggressive and frequently underrecognized neoplasms. *Mod. Pathol.* 2010; 23:781-9.

[83] Castilla MÁ, Moreno-Bueno G, Romero-Pérez L, De Vijver KV, Biscuola M, López-García MÁ, Prat J, Matías-Guiu X, Cano A, Oliva E, Palacios J. Micro-RNA signature of the epithelial-mesenchymal transition in endometrial carcinosarcoma. *J. Pathol.* 2011; 223:72-80.

[84] Romero-Pérez L, Castilla MÁ, López-García MÁ, Díaz-Martín J, Biscuola M, Ramiro-Fuentes S, Oliva E, Matias-Guiu X, Prat J, Cano A, Moreno-Bueno G, Palacios J. Molecular events in endometrial carcinosarcomas and the role of high mobility group AT-hook 2 in endometrial carcinogenesis. *Hum. Pathol.* 2013 44:244-54.

In: Endometrial Cancer
Editors: I. Diaz-Padilla, J. Garcia-Donas
ISBN: 978-1-63321-323-4

Chapter IV

Imaging Techniques for Staging of Endometrial Carcinoma

Manjiri Dighe*[*] *and Neeraj Lalwani
University of Washington Medical Center Department of Radiology,
Seattle, WA, US

Abstract

Endometrial carcinoma is the most common female pelvic malignancy and the seventh most common neoplasm worldwide. The highest incidence is endometrial carcinoma is seen in North America and Europe. Endometrial cancer is staged according to the International Federation of Gynecology and Obstetrics (FIGO) surgical system. Preoperative imaging of the disease can help in planning the optimal course of treatment since clinical estimation of disease stage can be inaccurate in more than 20%. Cross-sectional imaging, especially magnetic resonance imaging (MRI), may detect gross myometrial extension or extension of tumor to the surrounding lymph nodes, which can alter management and therefore help in preoperative surgical planning. This issue is increasingly relevant as less invasive surgical techniques, such as laparoscopic surgeries, are becoming more common for lower stage cancers. Several imaging techniques such as MRI,

[*] Corresponding author: Manjiri Dighe, MD, FSAR, Associate Professor, Section Chief of Body Imaging, University of Washington Medical Center Department of Radiology, Box No 357115 Seattle, WA 98195. Tel No: 206-598-0024. Fax No: 206-598-0252.

computed tomography, transvaginal ultrasound and Positron Emission Tomography have been used as tools for staging of endometrial cancer. Currently, MRI is the most widely used modality for preoperative planning. This article discusses the use of imaging techniques in diagnosis, staging, and detection of endometrial cancer and treatment of recurrent disease.

Introduction

Endometrial carcinoma (EC) is the most common gynecological malignancy and the seventh most common neoplasm worldwide. The highest incidence is endometrial carcinoma is seen in North America and Europe, and typically presents with abnormal uterine (intermenstrual or postmenopausal) bleeding in 75% to 90% of patients [1]. Endometrial carcinoma is a cancer predominantly seen in postmenopausal women and often detected early as patients present with vaginal bleeding [2]. However, currently, because of the increasing use of hormone replacement therapy, irregular vaginal bleeding in a postmenopausal woman may be overlooked, and investigation may be delayed. Because of early clinical symptoms, 75% of patients are diagnosed with early stage disease, with the peak incidence occurring around the sixth or seventh decade of life [3].

Advances in medicine have now made it possible for treatment to be more individualized (e.g. tissue typing). This underscores the need for comprehensive staging examination – one that can help identify patients appropriate for different therapies. In the case of gynecologic malignancies, the need for accurate staging is crucial, as a patient's best hope for cure is often the initial intervention. Even so, many women still are understaged, even by experienced gynecologic oncologists, because tumor deposits remain occult either because of location (e.g., under the hemidiaphragm) or because of their small size [4, 5]. Similarly, treatment for endometrial cancer relies on appropriate staging. The decision of whether or not to do lymph node sampling or a more modest surgery is directly related to depth of myometrial invasion. This chapter discusses the imaging protocol and describes interpretation models based on FIGO staging classifications to stage endometrial carcinoma.

FIGO Staging System (Revised)

The International Federation of Gynecology and Obstetrics (FIGO) staging system is the most widely accepted method for staging endometrial and cervical cancers [6]. The first FIGO staging system was created in 1958 and updated in 1988. Since that time, staging has changed considerably and data collection now allowed identification and analysis of specific prognostic factors in surgical-pathological staging. In the following years, surgical staging became routinely adopted by the great majority of institutions all over the world. Since Volume 23 of the FIGO Annual Report, the first data collection dealing with the surgical staging of endometrial cancer, over 42,000 patients with endometrial cancer have been reported. Because of this in-depth statistical analysis, the FIGO Committee could evaluate specific substages and prognosis. In Volume 26, surgical Stage IA G1, IB G1, IA G2, and IB G2 had a 5-year survival of 93.4%, 91.6%, 91.3%, and 93.4%, respectively [7]. These were not significantly different. In addition, these results were very similar in Volumes 23, 24, and 25.With this large database and follow-up, the Committee felt that some of these substages could be combined. This resulted in the revisions to the staging for endometrial cancer adopted in 2008 (Table 1). The 1988 Stage IA and IB have been combined so that now Stage IA involves the endometrium and/or less than one-half myometrial invasion and IB is equal to or greater than the outer one-half of the myometrium. The 3 grades still apply. The substages within Stage I have decreased from 9 to 6. In addition, Stage II no longer has a subset A and B. Involvement in the endocervical glandular portion of the cervix is now considered Stage I. The other area of note is that pelvic and para-aortic node involvement has been separated rather than combining them in a single substage. This seems to be reasonable since data would suggest that the prognosis is worse if the para-aortic nodes are involved. As a result, Stage IIIC is now categorized as IIIC1 (indicating positive pelvic nodes) and IIIC2 (indicating positive para-aortic nodes with or without positive pelvic nodes). This has significant implications in how staging is performed on the various imaging modalities.

Table 1. Revised FIGO classification

Stage			Revised FIGO staging (2008)		1988 FIGO Staging
I	Tumor confined to the corpus uteri.				
	IA		No or less than half myometrial invasion.		Tumor limited to the endometrium
	IB		Invasion equal to or more than half of the myometrium.		Invasion < 1/2 myometrium
				IC	Invasion > 1/2 myometrium
II	Tumor invades cervical stroma but does not extend beyond the uterus.				
				IIA	Endocervical glandular involvement
				IIB	Cervical stromal invasion
III	Local and/or regional spread of the tumor.				
	IIIA		Tumor invades the serosa of the corpus uteri and/or adnexae.		Tumor invades serosa and/or adnexa, and/or positive peritoneal cytology
	IIIB		Vaginal and/or parametrial involvement.		Vaginal metastases
	IIIC		Metastases to pelvic and/or para-aortic lymph nodes.		Metastases to pelvic and/or paraaortic lymph nodes
		IIIC1	Positive pelvic nodes.		
		IIIC2	Positive para-aortic lymph nodes with or without positive pelvic lymph nodes.		
IV	Tumor invades bladder and/or bowel mucosa, and/or distant metastases.				
IVA			Tumor invasion of bladder and/or bowel mucosa.		Tumor invasion of bladder and/or bowel mucosa
IVB			Distant metastases, including intra-abdominal metastases and/or inguinal lymph nodes.		Distant metastases including intraabdominal and/or inguinal lymph nodes

Adapted from FIGO Committee on Gynecologic Oncology (6).

Imaging Techniques

Endometrial cancer is surgically staged and imaging cannot replace surgical staging, however imaging may be valuable in multidisciplinary treatment planning. Accurate assessment by pre-treatment imaging can optimize surgical and non-surgical treatment particularly with regard to the use of pre-operative, neo-adjuvant therapy in advanced disease [8]. MR imaging is used to evaluate the depth of myometrial invasion and cervical invasion. The likelihood of lymphatic involvement is greater with greater myometrial penetration of tumor. CT or MR are used to assess nodal involvement [9, 10], however CT and MRI criteria for metastatic lymphadenopathy are based on size criteria. PET imaging has been shown to be more accurate in identifying metastatic lymph nodes, particularly in nodes considered normal by size criteria [11, 12].

Ultrasound

Even though transvaginal ultrasound is the imaging procedure of choice to evaluate patients with postmenopausal bleeding, the imaging features of endometrial carcinoma are non-specific, appearing as a thickened endometrium and ultrasound cannot reliably differentiate between benign proliferation, hyperplasia, polyps and cancer (figure 1). Transvaginal ultrasound can be used to evaluate the depth of myometrial invasion [13, 14]. A study by Akbayir et al. showed that TVS had a sensitivity, specificity, PPV, NPV and accuracy of 62%, 81%, 60%, 82%, and 75% respectively in predicting myometrial infiltration > 50% [15]. Gordon et al. in their study in 25 patients found that they could predict the depth of invasion correctly in 81.1% of cases when classified as none, superficial (less than 1/3rd), intermediate (middle third) and deep (outer third) [16]. They achieved sensitivity, specificity and accuracy of 75%, 75% and 76% respectively. Köchli et al. found sensitivity of TVS in predicting myometrial invasion of less than half of the uterine wall to be 100%, however for more than half, it was only 58%. In their study, overall accuracy was 80%, however they had a small number of patients in their study [17]. Factors that limit ultrasound TVS include distortion from multiple or large leiomyomas, adenomyosis, cavity hemorrhage, necrosis, and poor soft tissue contrast [18, 19].

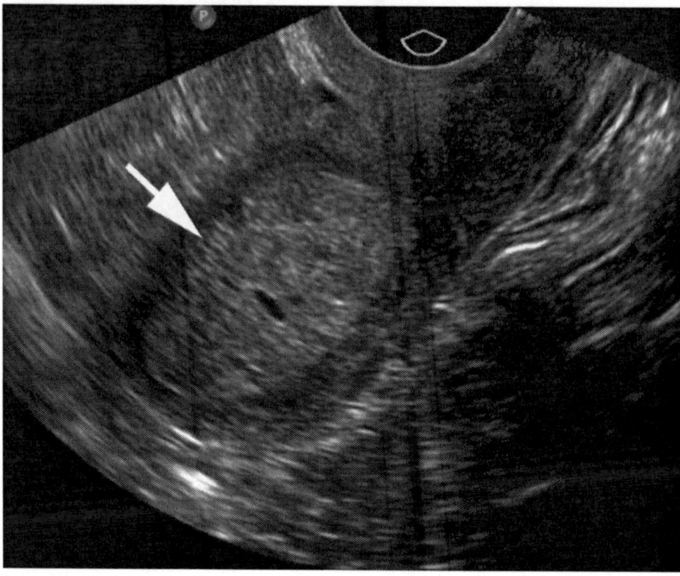

Figure 1. US showing a thickened endometrium measuring 2.3cm (arrow). This patient then had a biopsy of the endometrium which was positive for endometrial carcinoma.

Saline infusion sonohysterography (SIUS) may help to differentiate polyps, hyperplasia and carcinoma. This improves specificity of TVS in differentiating endoluminal masses from diffuse endometrial thickening. Takac in his study found that for superficial myometrial invasion, evaluation by TVS was accurate in 76.0% cases, and evaluation by SIUS was accurate in 72.0% of cases. For deep myometrial invasion, evaluation by TVS was accurate in 85.7% cases, and evaluation by SIUS was accurate in 96.4% of case [20]. However SIUS is an invasive procedure and the procedure itself may disseminate malignant cells into the peritoneal cavity through the fallopian tubes [21, 22].

Contrast enhanced sonography involves the use of ultrasound based contrast that act as blood pool markers and echo enhancers that sensitively reflect blood perfusion. Song et al. in their study found that the endometrial carcinomas started to enhance earlier than or at the same time as myometrium in 90.5% of women and the peak intensity, enhancement intensity, and rising rate were higher in endometrial lesion than normal myometrium. This allowed for easier recognition of the endometrial lesions [23]. Time intensity curves were calculated by the authors who showed a clear arrival time, rapid peak and decrease with return to the baseline level.

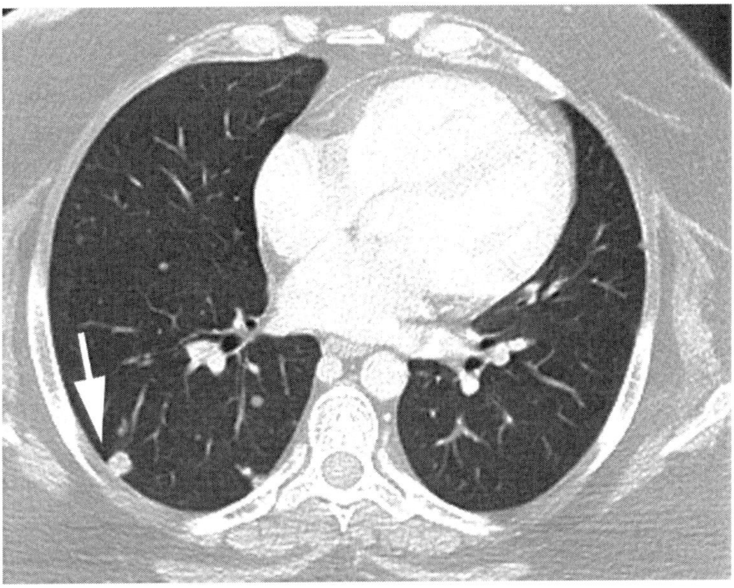

a

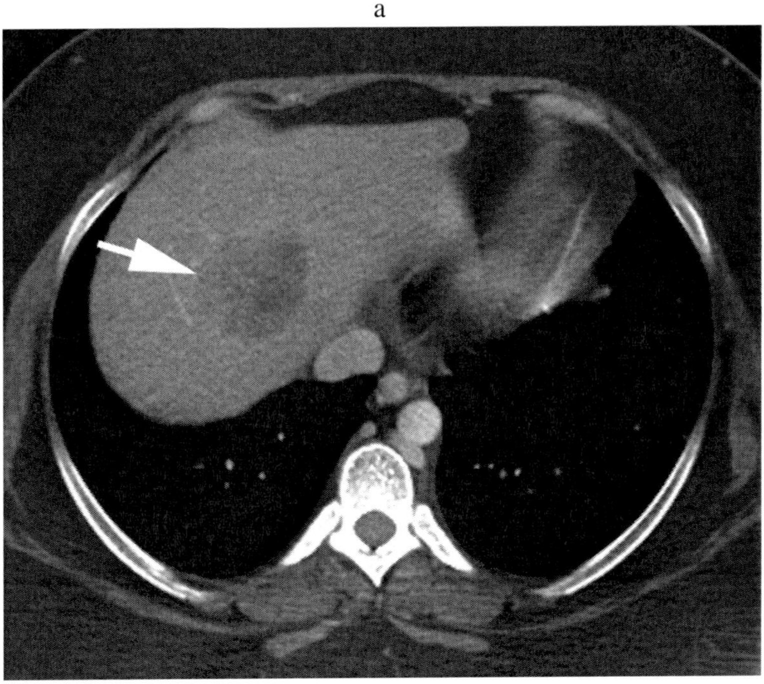

b

Figure 2. (Continued)

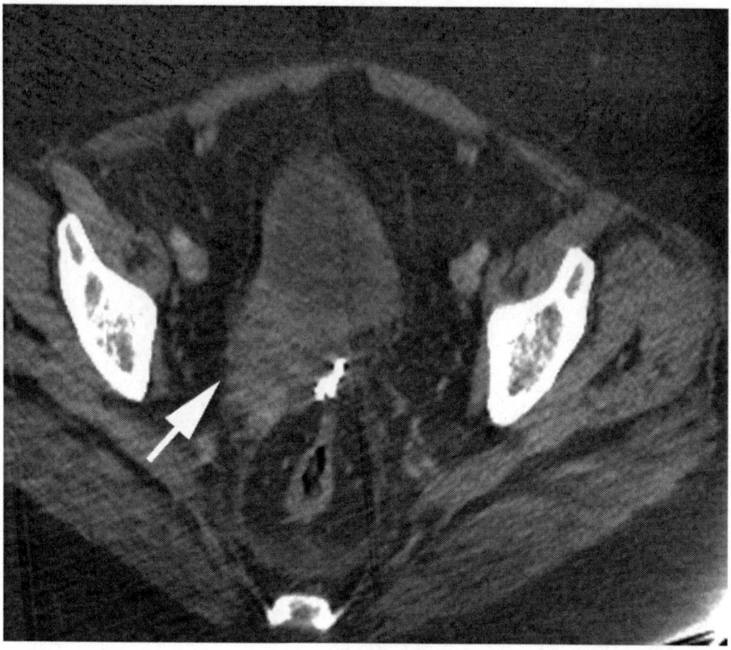

c

Figure 2. Computed Tomography in staging of endometrial carcinoma. Patient with proven endometrial carcinoma has metastases (arrows) to the lung (a), liver (b) and vaginal cuff (c).

Liu et al. evaluated the utility of contrast-enhanced sonography as an adjunct to conventional TVS for detecting endometrial carcinoma and defining the depth of myometrial invasion. They found that contrast-enhanced sonography contributed the most to tumor imaging in patients with a thin endometrium after endometrial biopsy because it enhanced the contrast between the tumor and tissue. The diagnostic accuracy of contrast-enhanced sonography for determining the myometrium infiltration depth in their study was 85.3% [24].

Limitation of contrast enhanced sonography includes the availability of the contrast agent and time-intensity curve can only be assessed when the probe is fixed during examination, and the analysis is performed offline after contrast-enhanced sonography is completed which precludes real time assessment.

Computed Tomography

CT is usually readily available and provides a rapid assessment and global overview of the abdomen and pelvis for distant metastases (figure 2). Soft tissue contrast resolution of CT is lower than that of MR imaging but spatial resolution is higher. CT has been extensively used to stage endometrial cancer, with overall accuracy for conventional CT ranging from 84–88% [25, 26]. Varpula et al. [27] and Kim et al. [28] reported an accuracy of 61% and 67% for CT, versus 89% and 83% for MRI in evaluating the depth of myometrial invasion in patients with endometrial carcinoma. Dore et al. [29] reported a 76% agreement between the CT findings and histopathologic results in predicting the depth of myometrial infiltration, and Hasumi et al. [30] assessed correctly the depth of myometrial invasion in all patients and the presence of cervical infiltration in 90% of cases. Hardesty et al. using a single-slice helical CT scanner reported a sensitivity of 83% and a specificity of 42% in evaluating the presence of deep myometrial invasion and a sensitivity of 25% and a specificity of 70% in the detection of cervical involvement, concluding that helical CT was much less accurate than MRI [31]. Evaluation of myometrial invasion by CT was initially hampered by imaging limited to the axial plane. In some cases the lie of the uterus was variable and usually not perpendicular to the axial plane as well. Current multidetector-row CT (MDCT) scanners have made thin slices, isotropic datasets, and reconstruction in multiple user-defined planes possible. Using multiplanar reconstructions and imaging 70 seconds after contrast injection on a 16-row MDCT scanner, the depth of myometrial invasion was correctly assessed in 18 of 21 patients with endometrial cancer [32].

Mri

Magnetic resonance (MR) imaging can accurately help assess the depth of myometrial invasion. MR imaging findings are also an important predictor of lymph node metastases. MR findings when combined with tumor grade and histology are also useful in selecting patients at low risk for recurrence [33]. Additional information from an MR imaging staging examination (e.g., uterine size, tumor volume, presence of ascites or adnexal disease) helps determine the surgical approach. Diffusion-weighted and dynamic multiphase contrast medium–enhanced MR imaging sequences have been shown to improve the accuracy of MR imaging in assessing the depth of myometrial invasion and can be used to assess tumor response to therapy and to differentiate tumor recurrence from post-treatment changes [34-36].

MRI Protocol

Patient Preparation

Patient preparation is essential to obtain good diagnostic quality examination in MRI. Due to the proximity of the bowel to the uterus, bowel motion frequently results in artifact over the regions of interest in the endometrium and cervix. Antiperistaltic agents such as glucagon or hyoscine butyl bromide (not available in the USA) may improve image quality [37]. Due to the short duration of action of an intravenous dose, antiperistaltic agents administered intramuscularly have relatively rapid absorption and the agent's length of action is approximately 30 minutes, which suits most MRI examinations [38]. Fasting for 4 to 6 hours before the examination and using an antiperistaltic drug reduce artifact from bowel motion. The patient should void approximately ½ to 1 hour prior to ensure that the bladder is only partially full since a full bladder may make the patient uncomfortable and an empty bladder will hamper adequate evaluation of any extension into the bladder [6].

Coils

To examine the pelvis effectively, a multichannel array coil is the preferred option. However in patients who are extremely obese, a body coil can be used and may provide equally good pelvic images. The use of a multichannel array coil also allows parallel imaging, which reduces scan time without a significant decline in the signal-to-noise ratio. Appropriate positioning of the patient in the coil allows coverage from the pelvic floor to the lower paraaortic lymph nodes helping to evaluate for nodal metastases as well.

Magnetic Resonance Imaging Sequences

T2-weighted sequences forms the mainstay for assessment of abnormalities of the pelvis including the uterine body and cervix. The intermediate signal intensity of an endometrial tumor is well delineated against the low signal intensity of the junctional zone or the inner cervical stroma. Orthogonal T2-weighted sequence imaging perpendicular to the uterine corpus may help in determining the depth of myometrial invasion and in delineating viable tumor in younger patients where the junctional zone is evident. T1-weighted images (T1WIs) supplement T2-weighted images (T2WIs) by detecting hemorrhage which are frequently seen in these patients as most of them have undergone endometrial biopsy before imaging.

Junctional zone is the landmark for determining the depth of myometrial invasion, however it is not always detectable in postmenopausal women. Therefore, the T2-weighted sagittal images may not provide adequate information, and T1-weighted fat-saturated 3-dimensional (3D) dynamic images provide a more accurate detection of myometrial and cervical invasion [9, 39, 40].

The use of dynamic contrast-enhanced imaging after the administration of intravenous gadolinium helps detect the depth of myometrial invasion and is especially useful when the zonal anatomy of the uterus is no longer evident or is disrupted. Primary tumors may appear isointense to normal uterine tissue on T1WIs and can have a variable T2 signal [9, 39, 41]. On gradient-echo T1-weighted dynamic imaging, high contrast is present between mildly enhancing tumor and the strongly enhancing subendometrial lining at 50 to 120 seconds after contrast injection [42]. The overall diagnostic performance of MRI for predicting depth of myometrial invasion is reported to be high, with high sensitivity (94%) but low specificity (50%) and a high negative predictive value (91%) [43]. Endometrial cancer can show early-arterial-phase enhancement and late gradual washout, whereas benign lesions and sarcomas generally enhance in the delayed phase, although this is not entirely specific [44]. Typically, T2WIs are less useful in predicting myometrial invasion [42]. Protocol used in our institution is illustrated in table 2.

Table 2. MR Imaging Technique for staging of Endometrial Carcinoma

Parameter	Axial T1W	Axial T2W	Sagittal T2W	Axial Oblique T2W	Axial DWI	Axial Multiphase DCE
Sequence	FSE	FRFSE	FRFSE	FRFSE	EPI	T1 SPIR
Repetition time (msec)	470	4500	4500	4500	5000	6.4
Echo time (msec)	16	85	85	85	85	2.1
No. of signals acquired	2	3	4	4	6	1
No. of dimensions	2	2	2	2	2	3
Section thickness (mm)	5	5	5	3	4.5	4.2
Gap (mm)	2.5	2.5	2.5	0.5	0	. . .
Matrix size	448 × 288	384 × 256	384 × 256	384 × 256	128 × 128	288 × 192
Field of view (mm)	240	240	240	220	240	320
Bandwidth (kHz)	31.25	31.25	41.67	41.67	. . .	83.33
No. of sections	20	20	21	26	21	24 per volume slab
b Value (sec/mm^2)	. . .	. . .	. . .	. . .	0, 400, 800	. . .
Timing relative to contrast medium injection	. . .	. . .	. . .	. . .	. . .	Preinjection, 30 sec, 60 sec, 3 min after injection
Acquisition time*	4 min 50 sec	3 min 10 sec	3 min 50 sec	4 min 30 sec	2 min 10 sec	17 sec

Note.—DCE = dynamic contrast-enhanced, DW = diffusion-weighted, EP = echoplanar, FRFSE = fast recovery fast spin-echo, FSE = fast spin-echo, SPIR = Spectral Presaturation with Inversion recovery, T1W = T1-weighted, T2W = T2-weighted.

*Varies depending on required coverage.

MRI In Primary Staging

The role of MRI in histologically proven endometrial carcinoma is to evaluate the depth of myometrial and cervical invasion. MRI has been acknowledged as a useful preoperative diagnostic tool with contrast enhanced MRI considered superior to ultrasound and CT for assessment of depth of myometrial and cervical invasion. Metastases to lymph nodes can also be evaluated with MRI. In addition, evaluation of depth of myometrial invasion can also help determine the need for lymph node dissection. These imaging findings can change patient management from potentially curative to palliative.

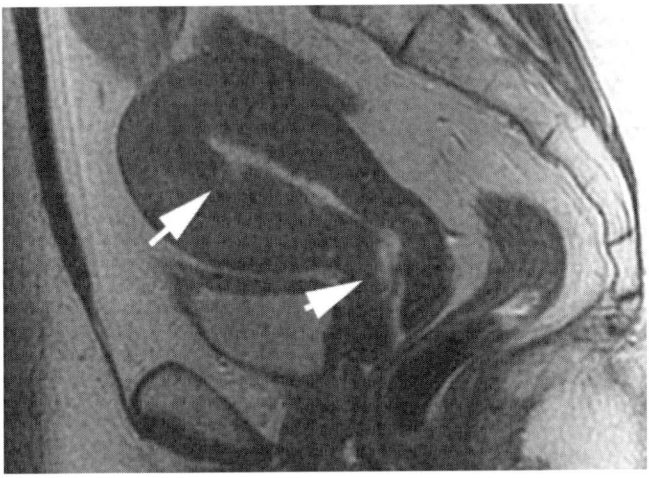

a

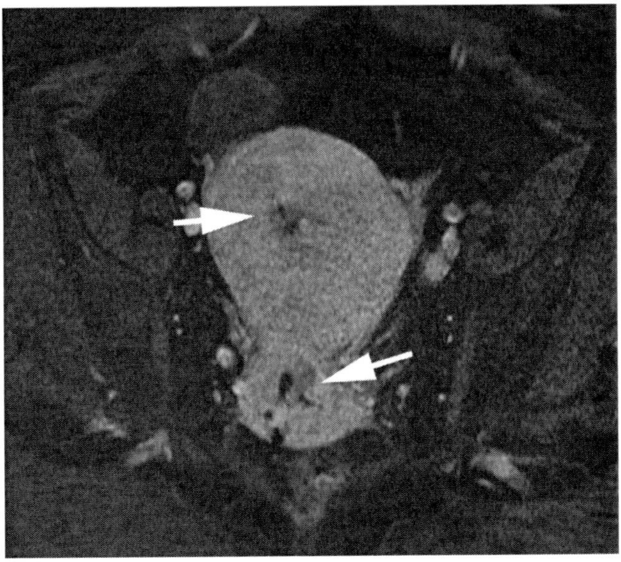

b

Figure 3. (Continued)

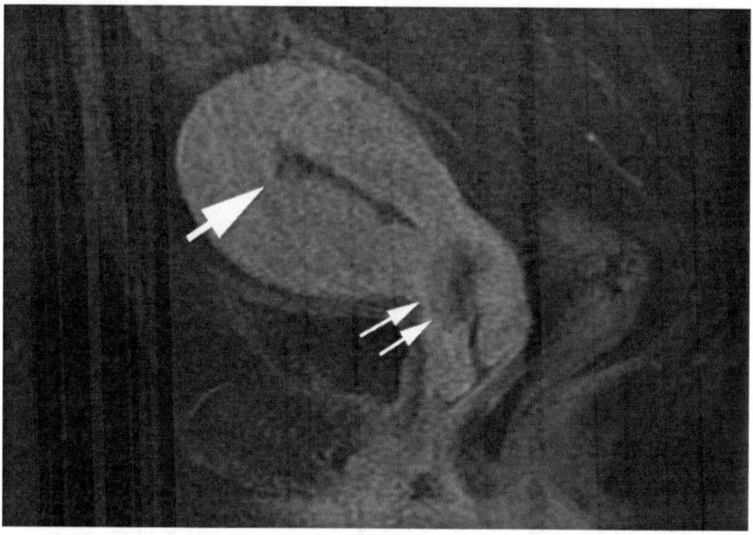

c

Figure 3. Stage 1b Endometrial carcinoma. Sagittal T2 weighted image (WI) (a) shows 2 areas of malignant involvement in the endometrium (arrows). Post contrast T1WIs (b) coronal and (c) sagittal show hypointense appearance of the endometrial carcinoma which is seen to extend greater than 50% of the myometrium in the lower region (double arrows).

Stage 0 and I Disease (Myometrium Invasion)

Stage 0 tumor (carcinoma in situ) disease usually does not show any abnormality in the endometrium one MRI. Tumor is seen to be confined to the endometrium or infiltrate less than 50% of the myometrium in stage 1A disease [18, 39, 41]. Infiltration of the myometrium is seen as discontinuity or disruption of the junctional zone (figure 3). In stage 1b disease, the tumor is seen to infiltrate greater than 50% of the myometrium with preservation of the outer myometrium. Coexistent adenomyosis can confound estimation of the depth of myometrial invasion as the endometrial-myometrial interface is irregular and T2WIs can overestimate/underestimate the depth of invasion (figure 4). This difficulty can be improved by using 3D dynamic imaging [44]. 3D dynamic imaging can improve sensitivity, specificity, positive predictive value, negative predictive value, and accuracy in detecting myometrial invasion, especially in postmenopausal women [44, 45]. Other pitfalls include due to polypoid tumors significantly compressing the myometrium, distension of the endometrial cavity by pyometria, presence of leiomyomata and poor tumor/myometrial contrast.

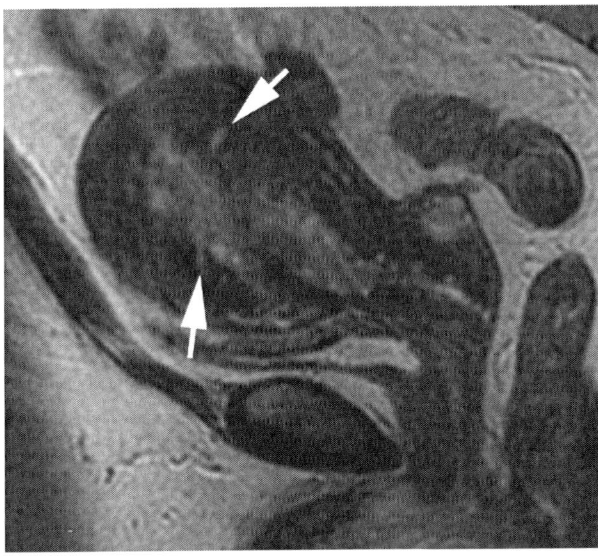

a

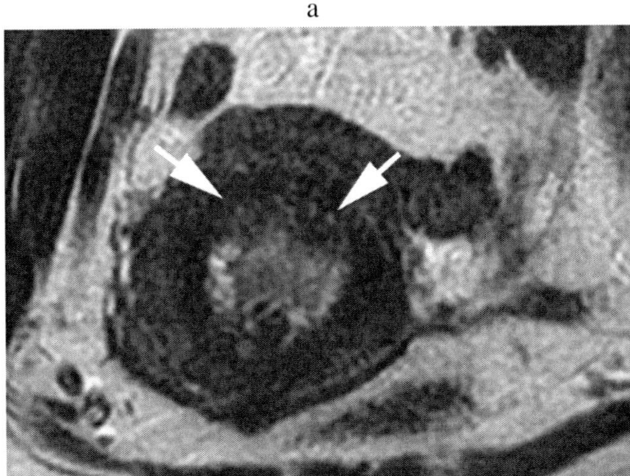

b

Figure 4. Stage 1 endometrial carcinoma with concomitant adenomyosis. Sagittal (a) and axial (b) T2WI shows hypointense appearance of the endometrial carcinoma however evaluation of extension is difficult due to concomitant adenomyosis seen as hyperintense areas in the junctional zone (arrows).

The literature is confusing regarding accuracy of MRI in assessing depth of invasion and staging as each study quotes a different parameters. Overall MRI has 87% sensitivity, 91% specificity, 89% accuracy, 97% positive predictive value, and 91% negative predictive value for the assessment of myometrial invasion in stages I disease [46]. Some studies have shown a significant improvement in accuracy of depth of myometrial invasion with dynamic contrast enhanced MRI over T2WIs, whereas other authors have not found any statistically significant difference. However these new techniques are felt to improve the specificity and PPV in differentiating deep myometrial invasion from superficial invasion and also level of diagnostic confidence [47, 48].

Stage II Disease (Cervical Invasion)

Stage II disease extends beyond the corpus into the cervix (figure 5). Normal cervical stroma demonstrates T2-weighted hypointensity and offers an exceptional contrast to the T2-weighted hyperintensity provided by the tumoral invasion [49]

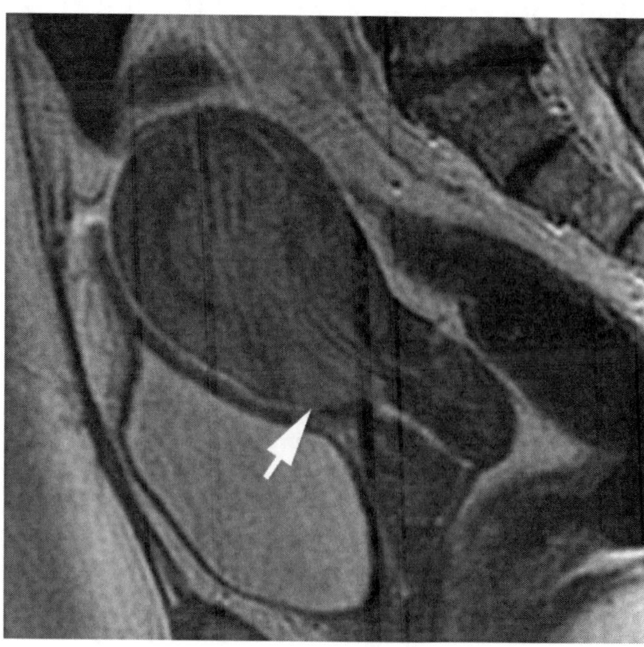

a

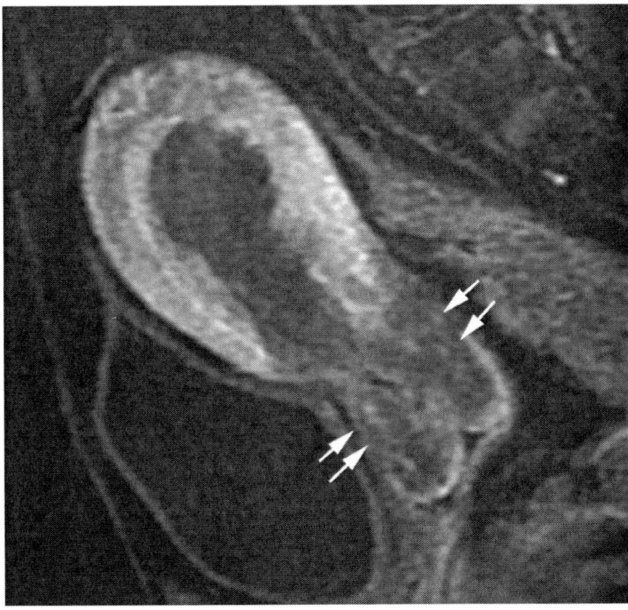

b

Figure 5. Stage II Endometrial carcinoma. Sagittal T2WI (a) shows hypointense endometrial carcinoma extending into the myometrium, however sagittal post contrast T1WI (b) shows hypoenhancing tumor (double arrows) extending into the cervix suggesting Stage II b disease.

In stage IIA disease, tumor extends into the endocervical canal from the endometrium and cause widening of the internal cervical os, with preservation of the fibrocervical stroma [3, 18, 39, 41]. In stage IIB disease the cervical stroma is involved which is seen as disruption of the high-signal ring-shaped cervical epithelium. This is well seen on 3D dynamic T1WIs specifically with a 180–240s delay [3]. The sensitivity, specificity, and diagnostic accuracy of cervical invasion have been reported to be 100%, 87%, and 90% on T2WIs, respectively; 100%, 95%, and 96% on postcontrast T1WIs, respectively; and 100%, 100%, and 100% on dynamic MRI, respectively [50]. The accuracy of sagittal T2WIs, thin section oblique axial T2WIs, sagittal contrast-enhanced T1WIs, and thin-section oblique axial contrast-enhanced T1WIs are 74.7%, 89.5%, 82.0%, and 95.5%, respectively [51]. MRI is superior to TVS and CT in predicting cervical stroma invasion but cannot reliably identify superficial mucosal invasion. A pitfall of imaging stage II disease is a polypoindal tumor protruding from the endometrial cavity into the endocervix [52].

Locally Advanced and Nodal Disease

Stage III disease extends outside the uterus but not beyond the true pelvis (figure 6). In stage IIIA, the outer myometrium is disrupted and irregular, with tumor invading the serosa or adnexa. Tumor extension to the adnexa may occur via the fallopian tubes, and surgery may reveal tumor cells in the peritoneum [18, 39, 41]. Extension to the vagina or parametrium results in loss of the normal low signal of the vaginal wall or as intermediate signal in the fat surrounding the uterus on T2WIs and is considered stage IIIB. Regional adenopathy indicates stage IIIC disease with metastasis to the pelvic nodes considered as stage IIIC1 disease and extension to the paraaortic nodes as stage IIIC2 disease. The location of nodal metastases corresponds to the drainage sites of the involved portions of the uterus. The middle and lower aspects of the uterus drain to the parametrium, paracervical and obturator lymph nodes. The upper corpus and fundus drain to common iliac and para-aortic lymph nodes. The inguinal nodes may be involved by spread along the round ligaments and rarely there is a direct para-aortic pathway [53]. There is no deifinite correation between the size of the tumor and risk of nodal disease as is seen in cerivical carcinoma.

MRI has 50% sensitivity, 95% specificity, 90% accuracy, 50% positive predictive value, and 95% negative predictive value for lymph node assessment [40]. Conventional MRI sequences cannot differentiate malignant from hyperplastic lymph nodes [41].

Numerous studies have suggested that a short axis size of more than 1 cm and necrosis can reliably predict lymph node involvement [41]. However, it has been shown that size criteria >10 mm in the shortest axis has low sensitivity (17%–80%) and high specificity (93%–100%). On the other hand, reducing the cut-off to 8 mm increases the sensitivity but decreases the specificity [43]. Sequences used for detection of lymph node metastases are axial T2-weighted, coronal T1-weighted, and fast imaging employing steady-state acquisition. Lymph node specific contrast agents like Ultrasmall superparamagnetic iron oxide particles (USPIOs) have been advocated but have not yet been approved for clinical use in the United States [54].

In stage IV disease, tumor extends beyond the true pelvis. In stage IVA disease, tumor involves the adjacent bowel, urinary bladder, or the rectum which is seen as loss of normal low T2 signal intensity of the bowel or the bladder wall [18].

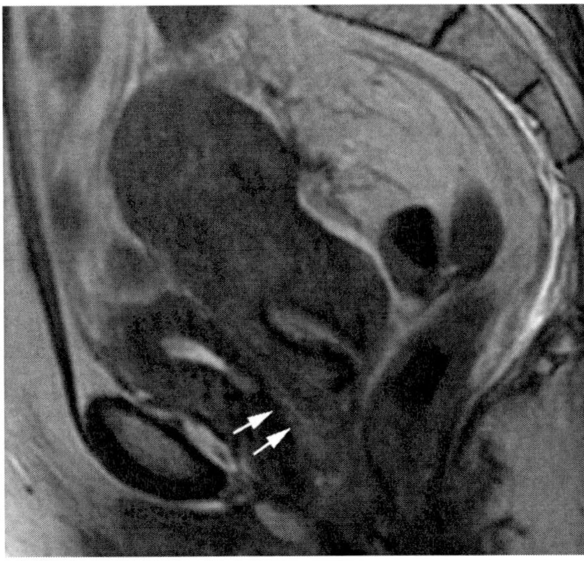

a

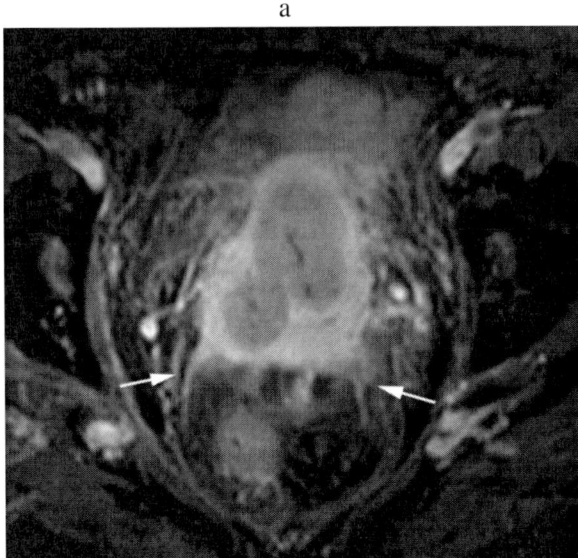

b

Figure 6. Stage 3 Endometrial carcinoma. Sagittal T2WI shows hypointense tumor extending into the vaginal wall (double arrows). Post contrast axial image shows the enhancement and thickening seen in the parametrium (arrows) suggesting extension of the tumor.

Metastatic Spread (Stage IVB Disease)

Distant metastases, nodal metastases, and peritoneal carcinomatosis suggest stage IVB disease. MRI has been reported to be superior to CT in the detection of peritoneal nodules greater than 1 cm and detection of peritoneal disease is improved by using dynamic fat-saturated T1-weighted contrast-enhanced images with gadolinium [18]. Patients with distant spread are more likely to have poorly differentiated/anaplastic cancers.

Recurrent Disease

MRI can be helpful in evaluation of recurrent disease. The most frequently observed sites of relapse are the lymph nodes, peritoneum, and the lung (figure 7). Recurrence can occur in the regional lymph nodes in descending order: paracervical/parametrial nodes followed by obturator, external, and internal iliac nodes. Secondary spread can be seen in the sacral, common iliac, inguinal, and paraaortic lymph nodes and in the tertiary nodes, including the peribronchial and supraclavicular nodal chains [55]. Recurrence within the vagina and the fallopian tube is less common [56]. The most common site for recurrent EC within the vagina is at the vaginal apex, and the tumor appears as a high-signal-intensity mass on the T2WIs [57, 58]. Metastases to the liver and the spleen are a significant predictor of poor outcome [59].

Diffusion-Weighted Imaging (DWI) in Endometrial Carcinoma

Diffusion-weighted imaging is a functional imaging technique which provides information about water mobility, tissue cellularity and integrity of cell membranes. As with other tumors, endometrial cancer exhibits impeded diffusion compared with surrounding tissue, manifesting as high signal intensity on diffusion-weighted MR images and low signal intensity on ADC maps, which provide a quantitative measure of water diffusion [60-63]. DWI images should always be reviewed with their corresponding ADC maps and other anatomic images to avoid pitfalls. These include T2 shine-through (apparent high signal intensity of a lesion due to the long T2) and impeded diffusion in areas of retained mucus in an obstructed endometrial canal.

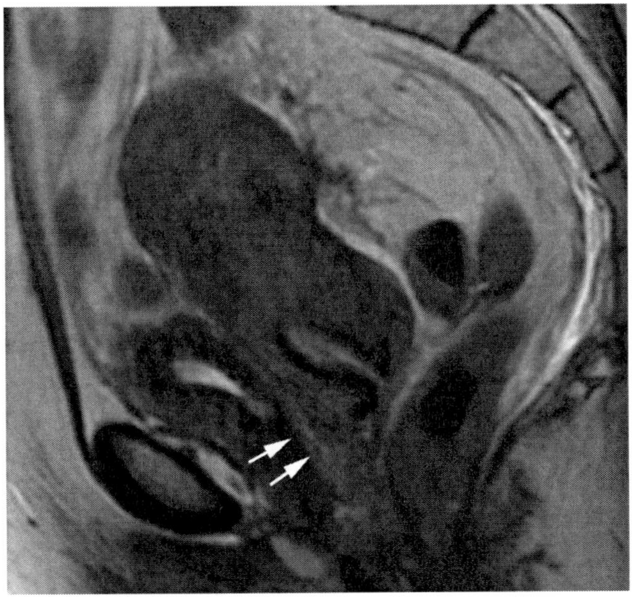

a

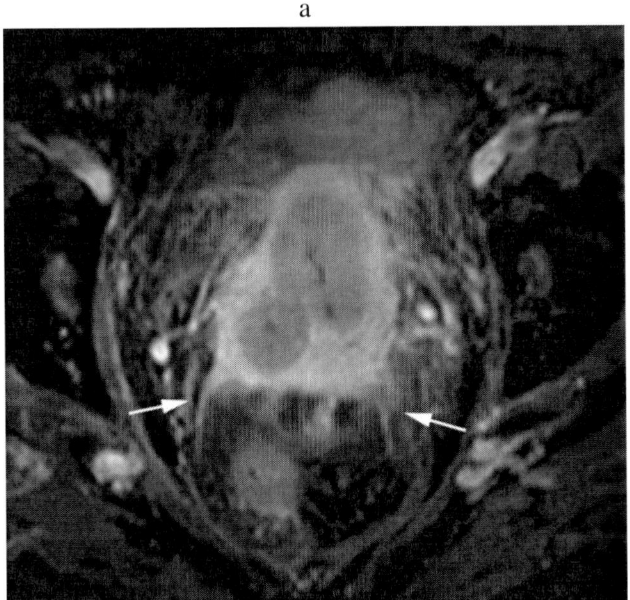

b

Figure 7. Recurrent disease. Follow up MRI in a patient with known endometrial carcinoma shows an enhancing lymph nodal mass in the right pelvis (arrows) on the post contrast axial (a) and coronal (b) images.

In a recent prospective study by Rechichi et al. [35], the staging accuracy of DW imaging was superior to that of dynamic contrast-enhanced MR imaging and had a higher level of interobserver agreement. The authors suggested that diffusion-weighted MR imaging could replace dynamic contrast-enhanced MR imaging for endometrial cancer staging, offering the potential advantages of reduced scanning time and obviation of the intravenous administration of gadolinium-based contrast medium [35]. DWI can also provide quantitative information in the form of ADC values. It has been revealed that metastatic lymph nodes demonstrate lower ADC values than the normal lymph nodes, and minimum ADC region values are more accurate than the mean values to confirm the suspicion of metastasis [35]. The cut-off value of 0.807 x 10−3mm^2/s, has shown higher sensitivity, specificity and overall accuracy [64].

However there are conflicting reports in the literature about the role of DWI in evaluation of lymph node metastases. Lin et al. [65] demonstrated that 3.0-T MR imaging had a greater sensitivity in the detection of nodal metastases in patients with endometrial carcinoma. The authors reported that ADC values for malignant nodes were significantly lower than those for benign nodes, and that the use of nodal ADC values combined with lymph node size yielded a sensitivity of 83% for assessing the presence of nodal malignancy [65]. In contrast, Nakai et al. [66] used 1.5-T MR imaging to evaluate nodal ADC values in gynecologic malignancies and were unable to differentiate benign from malignant lymph nodes. However, they did find that DWI MR imaging was useful in the detection of lymph nodes. Malignant tumors have significantly lower ADC values than benign lesions such as endometrial polyps and submucosal leiomyomas [63]. Tumor necrosis in poorly differentiated lesions, however, may also have high ADC values [60, 63].

Other techniques like MR perfusion and MR spectroscopy have been used in evaluation of endometrial carcinoma. MR perfusion is a variant of dynamic contrast-enhanced MRI, with repeated acquisitions of sequential images during the passage of a contrast agent through a tissue of interest. Postprocessing of the dynamic contrast-enhanced images with placement of a region of interest (ROI) enables plotting of signal intensity versus time graphs and measurements of maximum enhancement, peak enhancement, rate of peak enhancement, and signal enhancement ratios. MR perfusion is established as a promising technique to provide biomarkers and predictors of response to therapy for many tumour sites [67].

MR spectroscopy is a method to obtain biochemical information non-invasively from biological tissue. Within a defined volume of interest, signals may be registered from chemical nuclei within the body; the most commonly used nuclei are protons (hydrogen). Recently the scope of MR spectroscopy has expanded to include various organs, and has proved a valuable adjunct in the assessment of several types of cancers [67]. In endometrial carcinomas increased signals from choline [68], lipids [69], and lactate [68] within the tumour have been reported in small numbers of patients. These findings should be validated in larger studies to establish the typical pattern of biochemical markers in endometrial carcinomas. However future studies are needed to explore whether these biomarkers are relevant for the prediction of prognosis and therapeutic response in endometrial carcinomas.

PET/CT

Positron Emission Tomography has been used in oncology for approximately 3 decades with ^{18}F-fluoro-deoxyglucose (^{18}F-FDG) being the most common radiotracer used. ^{18}F-FDG is taken up by malignant cells but is also taken up by metabolically active normal tissues like brain, bowel, genitourinary tract, salivary glands ad lymphoid tissue. Inflammation and infection can also be metabolically active. The development of combined PET/computed tomography (CT) scanners allows the use of CT as the attenuation map to correct the FDG emission data. Accurate anatomic definition of areas of increased FDG update can be obtained by CT which allows for better differentiation of benign from malignant lesions yielding a more specific report.

Like other neoplasms, endometrial carcinoma demonstrates increased rate of glycolysis and takes up ^{18}F-FDG (figure 8). Nonmalignant physiologic causes like normal endometrium, cyclical abnormalities like oligomenorrhoea and hormonal therapy in postmenopausal patients can also cause uptake in the endometrium however the Standardized Uptake Values (SUV) in these etiologies is much lower than in endometrial carcinoma.

A study by Antonsen et al., found sensitivity, specificity, PPV, NPV, and accuracy for PET/CT to be 93%, 49%, 41%, 95% and 61% and for MRI to be 87%, 57%, 44%, 92%, and 66% for predicting myometrial invasion. For predicting cervical invasion, the values were 43%, 94%, 69%, 85% and 83%, respectively, for PET/CT and 33%, 95%, 60%, 85%, and 82%, respectively for

MRI. When comparing the diagnostic performance they found PET/CT and MRI to be comparable in predicting myometrial invasion [70].

Combined PET/CT is useful in the management of endometrial cancer, particularly in the pre-operative detection of pelvic and para-aortic metastatic lymphadenopathy [71-73]. Antonesen et al. also found that for lymph node metastases, the sensitivity, specificity, PPV, NPV, and accuracy were 74%, 93%, 59%, 96%, and 91% for PET/CT and 59%, 93%, 40%, 97% and 90% for MRI. For cervical invasion and lymph node metastases, however, PET/CT was the best [70].

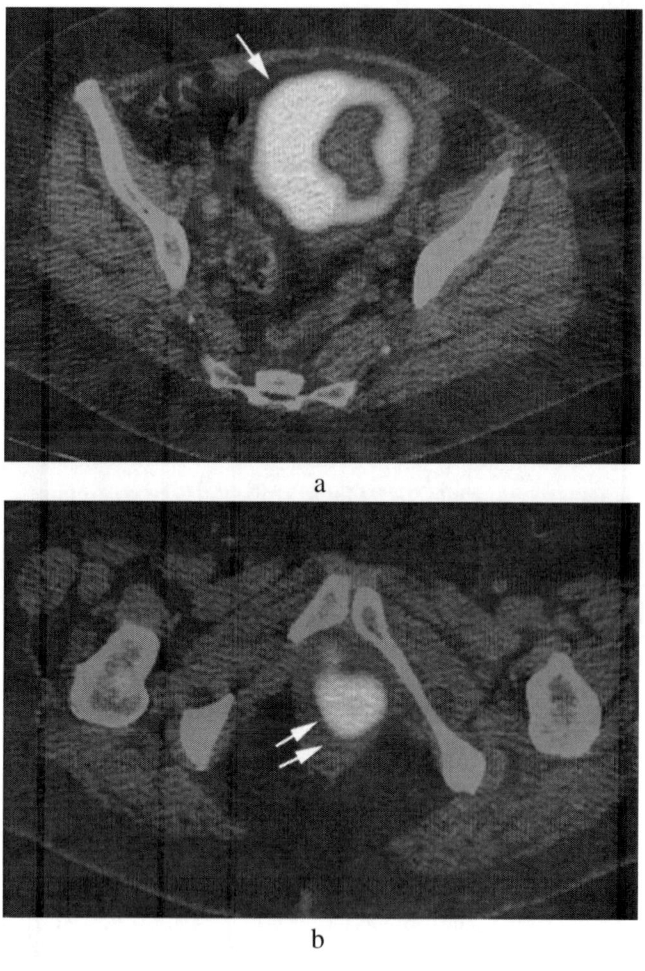

Figure 8. (Continued)

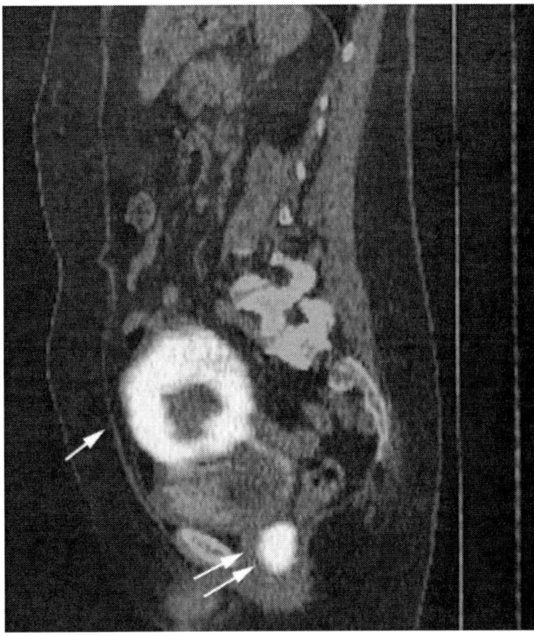

c

Figure 8. Positron Emission Tomography (PET) in endometrial carcinoma. Axial (a and b) and sagittal (b) images from a PET scan in a patient with known endometrial carcinoma show uptake in the primary mass in the uterus (arrow) and also uptake in a metastasis in the vaginal wall (double arrow) suggesting a stage III disease. Note patient did not have any other areas of uptake in the rest of the body as seen on sagittal image.

FDG PET has been used for detecting and evaluating recurrent endometrial cancer, with the advantage of imaging the entire body in a single study [73, 74]. Saga et al. found that PET\CT had a sensitivity of 100.0%, specificity of 88.2%, accuracy of 93.3% compared with combined conventional imaging which had a sensitivity of 84.6%, specificity of 85.7%, accuracy of 85.0% and tumor markers which had a sensitivity of 100.0%, specificity of 70.6% and accuracy of 83.3%. In their study, FDG-PET had no false-negative results and hence they suggested that FDG-PET can be used as a first-line examination in a patient's follow-up [73].

Belhocine in their study found that in 88% of their cases, the PET findings confirmed recurrence suggested by routine follow-up. In the remaining 12% of their cases, PET detected asymptomatic recurrences that were unsuspected at the control visits. Whole-body PET accurately localized the site of confirmed recurrences as being above and below the diaphragm in 50%, only below the diaphragm in 35% and only above the diaphragm in 15%. In one patient in their study, however, PET missed microscopic lung metastases shown on thoracic CT, and in three studies, metabolic imaging results were not confirmed. In 11 of 12 negative PET studies, no subsequent clinical or radiological recurrences were observed with a median follow-up of 10 months. Overall, the results of PET in their study agreed well with the final diagnosis (Cohen's kappa coefficient =0.78). In 9/26 patients (35%) with confirmed recurrences, the PET findings significantly altered the treatment choice by detecting either clinically or radiologically unsuspected distant metastases. The sensitivity, specificity, diagnostic accuracy and positive and negative predictive values of FDG PET imaging in the post-therapy surveillance of endometrial carcinomas in their study were 96%, 78%, 90%, 89% and 91%, respectively. The high likelihood ratio for a positive test result (4.5) and the low likelihood ratio for a negative test result (0.05) demonstrated the clinical utility of metabolic imaging in "ruling in" disease as well as "ruling out" recurrence. They concluded that whole-body FDG PET is useful in the post-therapy surveillance of endometrial cancers, both for the accurate localization of suspected recurrences and for the detection of asymptomatic recurrent disease [74].

Conclusion

Successful treatment of patients with endometrial carcinoma requires proper identification of the primary tumor and characterization of its local and regional spread. Endometrial carcinoma can be delineated on MRI, where T2WIs and dynamic 3D contrast-enhanced images provide excellent definition of the primary lesion and its extrauterine extension. However for a successful examination, good patient preparation, antiperistaltic agent use, and a scrupulous scanning technique is required. The multiplanar capabilities of MRI are invaluable for assessing disease margins and spread, and the 3D dynamic techniques offer the advantages of increased coverage and high spatial resolution. As MRI has excellent soft tissue contrast, it has become the standard for imaging uterine malignancies, providing a comprehensive assessment of disease before implementing potentially curative treatments such as surgery and radiotherapy. The clinical applications of PET/CT in patients with endometrial carcinoma are emerging. Further studies will be required to delineate its effect on outcome. Interpretation of PET/CT studies requires knowledge of physiologic endometrial activity and correlation with the patient's menstrual phase to avoid false positive interpretation of endometrial malignancy.

References

[1] Jemal A, Siegel R, Ward E, Hao Y, Xu J, Murray T, et al. Cancer statistics, 2008. *CA Cancer J Clin*. 2008;58:71-96.

[2] Daniels RV, McCuskey C. Abnormal vaginal bleeding in the nonpregnant patient. *Emerg Med Clin North Am*. 2003;21:751-72.

[3] Chaudhry S, Reinhold C, Guermazi A, Khalili I, Maheshwari S. Benign and malignant diseases of the endometrium. *Top Magn Reson Imaging*. 2003;14:339-57.

[4] Young RC, Decker DG, Wharton JT, Piver MS, Sindelar WF, Edwards BK, et al. Staging laparotomy in early ovarian cancer. *JAMA*. 1983;250:3072-6.

[5] McGowan L, Lesher LP, Norris HJ, Barnett M. Misstaging of ovarian cancer. *Obstet Gynecol*. 1985;65:568-72.

[6] Sala E, Wakely S, Senior E, Lomas D. MRI of malignant neoplasms of the uterine corpus and cervix. *AJR Am J Roentgenol*. 2007;188:1577-87.

[7] Creasman WT, Odicino F, Maisonneuve P, Quinn MA, Beller U, Benedet JL, et al. Carcinoma of the corpus uteri. FIGO 26th Annual Report on the Results of Treatment in Gynecological Cancer. *Int J Gynaecol Obstet*. 2006;95 Suppl 1:S105-43.

[8] Kinkel K, Kaji Y, Yu KK, Segal MR, Lu Y, Powell CB, et al. Radiologic staging in patients with endometrial cancer: a meta-analysis. *Radiology*. 1999;212:711-8.

[9] Frei KA, Kinkel K. Staging endometrial cancer: role of magnetic resonance imaging. *J Magn Reson Imaging*. 2001;13:850-5.

[10] Frei KA, Kinkel K, Bonél HM, Lu Y, Zaloudek C, Hricak H. Prediction of deep myometrial invasion in patients with endometrial cancer: clinical utility of contrast-enhanced MR imaging-a meta-analysis and Bayesian analysis. *Radiology*. 2000;216:444-9.

[11] Lerman H, Metser U, Grisaru D, Fishman A, Lievshitz G, Even-Sapir E. Normal and abnormal 18F-FDG endometrial and ovarian uptake in pre- and postmenopausal patients: assessment by PET/CT. *J Nucl Med*. 2004;45:266-71.

[12] Grisaru D, Almog B, Levine C, Metser U, Fishman A, Lerman H, et al. The diagnostic accuracy of 18F-fluorodeoxyglucose PET/CT in patients with gynecological malignancies. *Gynecol Oncol.* 2004;94:680-4.
[13] Dubinsky TJ, Parvey HR, Maklad N. The role of transvaginal sonography and endometrial biopsy in the evaluation of peri- and postmenopausal bleeding. *AJR Am J Roentgenol.* 1997;169:145-9.
[14] Grasel RP, Outwater EK, Siegelman ES, Capuzzi D, Parker L, Hussain SM. Endometrial polyps: MR imaging features and distinction from endometrial carcinoma. *Radiology.* 2000;214:47-52.
[15] Akbayir O, Corbacioglu A, Numanoglu C, Goksedef BP, Guraslan H, Akagunduz G, et al. Combined use of preoperative transvaginal ultrasonography and intraoperative gross examination in the assessment of myometrial invasion in endometrial carcinoma. *Eur J Obstet Gynecol Reprod Biol.* 2012;165:284-8.
[16] Gordon AN, Fleischer AC, Reed GW. Depth of myometrial invasion in endometrial cancer: preoperative assessment by transvaginal ultrasonography. *Gynecol Oncol.* 1990;39:321-7.
[17] Köchli OR, Bajka M, Schär G, Schmidt D, Haller U. [Measuring the death of invasion of endometrial carcinoma. Preoperative transvaginal ultrasound and correlation with intraoperative and histopathologic findings--a prospective study]. *Ultraschall Med.* 1995;16:8-11.
[18] Ascher SM, Reinhold C. Imaging of cancer of the endometrium. *Radiol Clin North Am.* 2002;40:563-76.
[19] Barwick TD, Rockall AG, Barton DP, Sohaib SA. Imaging of endometrial adenocarcinoma. *Clin Radiol.* 2006;61:545-55.
[20] Takac I. Transvaginal ultrasonography with and without saline infusion in assessment of myometrial invasion of endometrial cancer. *J Ultrasound Med.* 2007;26:949-55; quiz 56-7.
[21] Akin O, Mironov S, Pandit-Taskar N, Hann LE. Imaging of uterine cancer. *Radiol Clin North Am.* 2007;45:167-82.
[22] Dessole S, Rubattu G, Farina M, Capobianco G, Cherchi PL, Tanda F, et al. Risks and usefulness of sonohysterography in patients with endometrial carcinoma. *Am J Obstet Gynecol.* 2006;194:362-8.
[23] Song Y, Yang J, Liu Z, Shen K. Preoperative evaluation of endometrial carcinoma by contrast-enhanced ultrasonography. *BJOG.* 2009;116:294-8; discussion 8-9.
[24] Liu ZZ, Jiang YX, Dai Q, Yang M, Zhu QL, Zhao DC, et al. Imaging of endometrial carcinoma using contrast-enhanced sonography. *J Ultrasound Med.* 2011;30:1519-27.

[25] Walsh JW, Goplerud DR. Computed tomography of primary, persistent, and recurrent endometrial malignancy. *AJR Am J Roentgenol.* 1982;139:1149-54.

[26] Balfe DM, Van Dyke J, Lee JK, Weyman PJ, McClennan BL. Computed tomography in malignant endometrial neoplasms. *J Comput Assist Tomogr.* 1983;7:677-81.

[27] Varpula MJ, Klemi PJ. Staging of uterine endometrial carcinoma with ultra-low field (0.02 T) MRI: a comparative study with CT. *J Comput Assist Tomogr.* 1993;17:641-7.

[28] Kim SH, Kim HD, Song YS, Kang SB, Lee HP. Detection of deep myometrial invasion in endometrial carcinoma: comparison of transvaginal ultrasound, CT, and MRI. *J Comput Assist Tomogr.* 1995;19:766-72.

[29] Dore R, Moro G, D'Andrea F, La Fianza A, Franchi M, Bolis PF. CT evaluation of myometrium invasion in endometrial carcinoma. *J Comput Assist Tomogr.* 1987;11:282-9.

[30] Hasumi K, Matsuzawa M, Chen HF, Takahashi M, Sakura M. Computed tomography in the evaluation and treatment of endometrial carcinoma. *Cancer.* 1982;50:904-8.

[31] Hardesty LA, Sumkin JH, Hakim C, Johns C, Nath M. The ability of helical CT to preoperatively stage endometrial carcinoma. *AJR Am J Roentgenol.* 2001;176:603-6.

[32] Tsili AC, Tsampoulas C, Dalkalitsis N, Stefanou D, Paraskevaidis E, Efremidis SC. Local staging of endometrial carcinoma: role of multidetector CT. *Eur Radiol.* 2008;18:1043-8.

[33] Todo Y, Kato H, Kaneuchi M, Watari H, Takeda M, Sakuragi N. Survival effect of para-aortic lymphadenectomy in endometrial cancer (SEPAL study): a retrospective cohort analysis. *Lancet.* 2010;375:1165-72.

[34] Sala E, Rockall A, Rangarajan D, Kubik-Huch RA. The role of dynamic contrast-enhanced and diffusion weighted magnetic resonance imaging in the female pelvis. *Eur J Radiol.* 2010;76:367-85.

[35] Rechichi G, Galimberti S, Signorelli M, Perego P, Valsecchi MG, Sironi S. Myometrial invasion in endometrial cancer: diagnostic performance of diffusion-weighted MR imaging at 1.5-T. *Eur Radiol.* 2010;20:754-62.

[36] Sala E, Crawford R, Senior E, Shaw A, Simcock B, Vrotsou K, et al. Added value of dynamic contrast-enhanced magnetic resonance imaging

in predicting advanced stage disease in patients with endometrial carcinoma. *Int J Gynecol Cancer.* 2009;19:141-6.

[37] Martí-Bonmatí L, Graells M, Ronchera-Oms CL. Reduction of peristaltic artifacts on magnetic resonance imaging of the abdomen: a comparative evaluation of three drugs. *Abdom Imaging.* 1996;21:309-13.

[38] Dosdá R, Martí-Bonmatí L, Ronchera-Oms CL, Mollá E, Arana E. Effect of subcutaneous butylscopolamine administration in the reduction of peristaltic artifacts in 1.5-T MR fast abdominal examinations. *Eur Radiol.* 2003;13:294-8.

[39] Ascher SM, Takahama J, Jha RC. Staging of gynecologic malignancies. *Top Magn Reson Imaging.* 2001;12:105-29.

[40] Manfredi R, Mirk P, Maresca G, Margariti PA, Testa A, Zannoni GF, et al. Local-regional staging of endometrial carcinoma: role of MR imaging in surgical planning. *Radiology.* 2004;231:372-8.

[41] Manfredi R, Gui B, Maresca G, Fanfani F, Bonomo L. Endometrial cancer: magnetic resonance imaging. *Abdom Imaging.* 2005;30:626-36.

[42] Kinkel K. Pitfalls in staging uterine neoplasm with imaging: a review. *Abdom Imaging.* 2006;31:164-73.

[43] Rockall AG, Meroni R, Sohaib SA, Reynolds K, Alexander-Sefre F, Shepherd JH, et al. Evaluation of endometrial carcinoma on magnetic resonance imaging. *Int J Gynecol Cancer.* 2007;17:188-96.

[44] Utsunomiya D, Notsute S, Hayashida Y, Lwakatare F, Katabuchi H, Okamura H, et al. Endometrial carcinoma in adenomyosis: assessment of myometrial invasion on T2-weighted spin-echo and gadolinium-enhanced T1-weighted images. *AJR Am J Roentgenol.* 2004;182:399-404.

[45] Saez F, Urresola A, Larena JA, Martín JI, Pijuán JI, Schneider J, et al. Endometrial carcinoma: assessment of myometrial invasion with plain and gadolinium-enhanced MR imaging. *J Magn Reson Imaging.* 2000;12:460-6.

[46] Nakao Y, Yokoyama M, Hara K, Koyamatsu Y, Yasunaga M, Araki Y, et al. MR imaging in endometrial carcinoma as a diagnostic tool for the absence of myometrial invasion. *Gynecol Oncol.* 2006;102:343-7.

[47] Savci G, Ozyaman T, Tutar M, Bilgin T, Erol O, Tuncel E. Assessment of depth of myometrial invasion by endometrial carcinoma: comparison of T2-weighted SE and contrast-enhanced dynamic GRE MR imaging. *Eur Radiol.* 1998;8:218-23.

[48] Seki H, Kimura M, Sakai K. Myometrial invasion of endometrial carcinoma: assessment with dynamic MR and contrast-enhanced T1-weighted images. *Clin Radiol.* 1997;52:18-23.
[49] Haldorsen IS, Salvesen HB. Staging of endometrial carcinomas with MRI using traditional and novel MRI techniques. *Clin Radiol.* 2012;67:2-12.
[50] Murakami T, Kurachi H, Nakamura H, Tsuda K, Miyake A, Tomoda K, et al. Cervical invasion of endometrial carcinoma--evaluation by parasagittal MR imaging. *Acta Radiol.* 1995;36:248-53.
[51] Shibutani O, Joja I, Shiraiwa M, Asakawa T, Miyagi Y, Kudo T, et al. Endometrial carcinoma: efficacy of thin-section oblique axial MR images for evaluating cervical invasion. *Abdom Imaging.* 1999;24:520-6.
[52] Toki T, Oka K, Nakayama K, Oguchi O, Fujii S. A comparative study of pre-operative procedures to assess cervical invasion by endometrial carcinoma. *Br J Obstet Gynaecol.* 1998;105:512-6.
[53] Creutzberg CL, van Putten WL, Koper PC, Lybeert ML, Jobsen JJ, Wárlám-Rodenhuis CC, et al. Surgery and postoperative radiotherapy versus surgery alone for patients with stage-1 endometrial carcinoma: multicentre randomised trial. PORTEC Study Group. Post Operative Radiation Therapy in Endometrial Carcinoma. *Lancet.* 2000;355: 1404-11.
[54] Rockall AG, Sohaib SA, Harisinghani MG, Babar SA, Singh N, Jeyarajah AR, et al. Diagnostic performance of nanoparticle-enhanced magnetic resonance imaging in the diagnosis of lymph node metastases in patients with endometrial and cervical cancer. *J Clin Oncol.* 2005;23:2813-21.
[55] Jeong YY, Kang HK, Chung TW, Seo JJ, Park JG. Uterine cervical carcinoma after therapy: CT and MR imaging findings. *Radiographics.* 2003;23:969-81; discussion 81.
[56] Barakat RR, Goldman NA, Patel DA, Venkatraman ES, Curtin JP. Pelvic exenteration for recurrent endometrial cancer. *Gynecol Oncol.* 1999;75:99-102.
[57] Viswanathan AN, Cormack R, Holloway CL, Tanaka C, O'Farrell D, Devlin PM, et al. Magnetic resonance-guided interstitial therapy for vaginal recurrence of endometrial cancer. *Int J Radiat Oncol Biol Phys.* 2006;66:91-9.
[58] Sugimura K, Okizuka H. Postsurgical pelvis: treatment follow-up. *Radiol Clin North Am.* 2002;40:659-80, viii.

[59] Sohaib SA, Houghton SL, Meroni R, Rockall AG, Blake P, Reznek RH. Recurrent endometrial cancer: patterns of recurrent disease and assessment of prognosis. *Clin Radiol*. 2007;62:28-34; discussion 5-6.

[60] Tamai K, Koyama T, Saga T, Umeoka S, Mikami Y, Fujii S, et al. Diffusion-weighted MR imaging of uterine endometrial cancer. *J Magn Reson Imaging*. 2007;26:682-7.

[61] Fujii S, Matsusue E, Kigawa J, Sato S, Kanasaki Y, Nakanishi J, et al. Diagnostic accuracy of the apparent diffusion coefficient in differentiating benign from malignant uterine endometrial cavity lesions: initial results. *Eur Radiol*. 2008;18:384-9.

[62] Lin G, Ng KK, Chang CJ, Wang JJ, Ho KC, Yen TC, et al. Myometrial invasion in endometrial cancer: diagnostic accuracy of diffusion-weighted 3.0-T MR imaging--initial experience. *Radiology*. 2009;250:784-92.

[63] Shen SH, Chiou YY, Wang JH, Yen MS, Lee RC, Lai CR, et al. Diffusion-weighted single-shot echo-planar imaging with parallel technique in assessment of endometrial cancer. *AJR Am J Roentgenol*. 2008;190:481-8.

[64] Nagar H, Dobbs S, McClelland HR, Price J, McCluggage WG, Grey A. The diagnostic accuracy of magnetic resonance imaging in detecting cervical involvement in endometrial cancer. *Gynecol Oncol*. 2006;103:431-4.

[65] Lin G, Ho KC, Wang JJ, Ng KK, Wai YY, Chen YT, et al. Detection of lymph node metastasis in cervical and uterine cancers by diffusion-weighted magnetic resonance imaging at 3T. *J Magn Reson Imaging*. 2008;28:128-35.

[66] Nakai G, Matsuki M, Inada Y, Tatsugami F, Tanikake M, Narabayashi I, et al. Detection and evaluation of pelvic lymph nodes in patients with gynecologic malignancies using body diffusion-weighted magnetic resonance imaging. *J Comput Assist Tomogr*. 2008;32:764-8.

[67] Harry VN, Semple SI, Parkin DE, Gilbert FJ. Use of new imaging techniques to predict tumour response to therapy. *Lancet Oncol*. 2010;11:92-102.

[68] Okada T, Harada M, Matsuzaki K, Nishitani H, Aono T. Evaluation of female intrapelvic tumors by clinical proton MR spectroscopy. *J Magn Reson Imaging*. 2001;13:912-7.

[69] Celik O, Hascalik S, Sarac K, Meydanli MM, Alkan A, Mizrak B. Magnetic resonance spectroscopy of premalignant and malignant

endometrial disorders: a feasibility of in vivo study. *Eur J Obstet Gynecol Reprod Biol.* 2005;118:241-5.

[70] Antonsen SL, Jensen LN, Loft A, Berthelsen AK, Costa J, Tabor A, et al. MRI, PET/CT and ultrasound in the preoperative staging of endometrial cancer - a multicenter prospective comparative study. *Gynecol Oncol.* 2013;128:300-8.

[71] Yen TC, Lai CH. Positron emission tomography in gynecologic cancer. *Semin Nucl Med.* 2006;36:93-104.

[72] Horowitz NS, Dehdashti F, Herzog TJ, Rader JS, Powell MA, Gibb RK, et al. Prospective evaluation of FDG-PET for detecting pelvic and para-aortic lymph node metastasis in uterine corpus cancer. *Gynecol Oncol.* 2004;95:546-51.

[73] Saga T, Higashi T, Ishimori T, Mamede M, Nakamoto Y, Mukai T, et al. Clinical value of FDG-PET in the follow up of post-operative patients with endometrial cancer. *Ann Nucl Med.* 2003;17:197-203.

[74] Belhocine T, De Barsy C, Hustinx R, Willems-Foidart J. Usefulness of (18)F-FDG PET in the post-therapy surveillance of endometrial carcinoma. *Eur J Nucl Med Mol Imaging.* 2002;29:1132-9.

In: Endometrial Cancer
Editors: I. Diaz-Padilla, J. Garcia-Donas
ISBN: 978-1-63321-323-4

Chapter V

New Surgical Approaches to Early-Stage Endometrial Cancer

Stefano Palomba*[*], *Vincenzo Dario Mandato and Giovanni Battista La Sala
Academic Department of Obstetrics & Gynecology, Arcispedale S. Maria Nuova of Reggio Emilia, IRCCS,
University of Modena & Reggio Emilia, Italy

Abstract

Endometrial cancer (EC) is the most common gynecologic malignancy in developed countries with an increasing incidence. It is usually diagnosed at early stage and surgical treatment generally yield excellent survival outcomes. Standard surgical treatment for early stage EC includes peritoneal washing, total abdominal hysterectomy and bilateral salpingo-oophorectomy with or without pelvic and paraaortic lymphadenectomy. However, the lack of univocal data on the value of peritoneal washing, pelvic/paraaortic nodes resection and type II radical hysterectomy in early stage EC had simplified the use of several surgical approaches. Actually, the minimally invasive techniques are widely accepted by many authors for treating early stage EC, and the classical

[*] Correspondig Author: Stefano Palomba - Academic Department of Obstetrics & Gynecology, Arcispedale S. Maria Nuova of Reggio Emilia, IRCCS, University of Modena & Reggio Emilia, Via Risorgimento 80 - 42123 Reggio Emilia – Italy. Email: stefanopalomba@tin.

laparoscopic one should be considered the gold standard. Further techniques include the vaginal surgery, the robotic, the single port and micro/minilaparoscopic approaches. Fertility sparing surgery is also a potential approach for younger patients in reproductive age.

Introduction

Endometrial cancer (EC) is the most common gynecological malignancy in developed countries and the sixth most common malignancy of the female genital tract worldwide. Its incidence has increased due to longer life expectancy, increased obesity, and an increase in the use of tamoxifen to treat breast cancer women [1-4]. In a variable but very high proportion of cases, EC is diagnosed at early stage so its treatment generally yield excellent survival outcomes [5].

The definition of "early stage" EC refer generally to stage I according to International Federation of Gynecology and Obstetrics (FIGO) classification [6]. According to FIGO classification, cancer is in the endometrium only or less than halfway through the myometrium (stage IA) or it has spread halfway or more into the myometrium (stage IB) [6]. Moreover, in consideration of the recent updating of the FIGO classification and of the recent data on the role of surgical treatment in stage I and II EC, some authors consider an "early stage EC" all cancers without spread outside the uterus. In this view, also cancers with spread into connective tissue of the cervix (stage II) are included.

Because EC has a good overall cure rate and it is thought to be easily cured, in most geographical areas the majority of women are managed by generalist gynecologists rather than care being centralized to gynecologic oncology units. However, this results in a lack of staging and adequate procedures with a possible impact in quality of assistance [7].

All early stage ECs are not the same disease. Several factors can impact the prognosis of EC patients. High risk of recurrence in apparent early stage disease depends from histological subtype, grading, myometrial invasion, lymphovascular space invasion (LVSI), lymph node metastases and tumor diameter [8]. Following criteria adopted in the main randomized clinical trials (RCTs) available in literature [9-11], in the clinical practice early stage EC are subdivided into three risk categories: low risk, including stage IA, grading G1 and G2, and with endometrioid type; intermediate risk, including stage IA, grading G3, endometrioid type, and stage IB, grading G1 and G2, with endometrioid type; and high risk: including stage IB, grading G3, with endometrioid type, and all stages with non-endometrioid type. Other clinical characteristics, such as the patient's age, have been also reported as risk factors and indentify intermediate/high risk patients. Specifically, a cut-off age of 60 years without further risk factor [9], 50 years with two risk factors, or 70 without any risk factor [10] have been considered as criteria to consider an EC at intermediate/high risk [11].

Traditionally, standard surgical treatment for early stage EC includes peritoneal washing, total hysterectomy (TH) and bilateral salpingo-oophorectomy.

It is well know that definitive histologic grading, myometrial invasion and lymph node involvement differ in a substantial rate from intraoperative gross assessment (up to 15%) and frozen section results (up to 25%) [12,13], and, hence, definitive stage and treatment can be defined only after surgery. However, several controversies in the management of early stage EC have make possible the use of several surgical approaches, both demolitive and fertility-sparing, before experimented in the feasibility studies and then proposed in the clinical practice.

In the current chapter we will discuss the main concerns in surgical staging of early stage EC, the different surgical approaches for treating early stage EC and the fertility-sparing surgical techniques.

Main Concerns in Surgical Staging

As already stated above, the staging extension can influence significantly the choice of surgical approach in the clinical practice. To this regard, poor consensus there is regarding the peritoneal cytology (PC) results [14-28], and the role of radical hysterectomy (RH) [29-31] and of pelvic (PEL) and of paraaortic (PAL) lymphadenectomy [32-34].

Peritoneal Cytology

In the 2009 FIGO staging for EC, the evaluation of the PC was formally omitted because the presence of positive cells in peritoneal cavity was considered controversial as independent negative prognostic factor. Positive PC is not an independent negative prognostic indicator but potentiates other adverse prognostic indicators, especially for advanced stage EC [14-28].

Positive PC is common in patients with grading 3, extrauterine extension, deep myometrial invasion, or positive pelvic or para-aortic nodes [14-20]. An higher risk of recurrence was observed in EC patients with positive washings in comparison with negative washings (29.1 vs. 10.5%) [21], but 68% of recurrences with positive washings, the recurrences were outside the peritoneal cavity, even if the relative risk (RR) of death for patients with positive PC was 3 times higher [22]. In case of extrauterine disease spread, positive PC findings decreased the survival rate from 73% to 13% at 5 years and all recurrences were at distant sites [20].

In early stage EC, i.e. FIGO stage I, positive PC was detected in 8.3%, 12.1%, and 15.9% for grades 1, 2, and 3 histologic types, respectively [23]. After stratification for myometrial invasion, positive PC was observed in 7.6% and 17.2% of the cases with superficial and deep invasion, respectively [46]. In addition, positive PC did not influence survival when the disease was confined to the uterus (FIGO stage I and II EC) [20].

Radical (TYPE II) Hysterectomy

In 2009, an Italian multicenter RCT [29] compared the RH (Piver-Rutledge class II) to the standard extrafascial TH (Piver-Rutledge class I) in 520 patients with stage I EC having as primary endpoint the overall survival (OS) and as secondary the locoregional recurrences. Pathological analysis controlled the quality of the surgeries. Two arms resulted similar in 5-year disease-free survival (DFS) and OS (87.7 and 88.9% in the class I arm and 89.7 and 92.2% in the class II arm, respectively), risk for recurrence (OR 0.91; 95% CI, 0.55-1.51), and for death [hazard ratio (HR) 0.77; 95% CI, 0.44-1.33].

In the new FIGO staging system for EC [6], it is not need to distinguish between epithelial involvement and stromal invasion of the cervix. In fact, there is no difference in OS in EC patients sub-grouped according to superficial or deep cervical invasion [29].

However, RH is traditionally recommended for EC with suspected cervical involvement (FIGO stage II EC) in order to reduce the vaginal and pelvic recurrences (~5-20% of cases) that can be only controlled by radiotherapy. Furthermore, the efficacy of the surgical procedure has not been confirmed.

In a wide cohort study on a total 1577 EC patients, 1198 subjects who underwent simple TH were compared with other 379 women who underwent

RH. RH had no effect on survival even if patients who did not receive postoperative radiotherapy had a OS lower than those who underwent adjuvant radiotherapy, and this benefit was most pronounced in women who underwent RH [31].

More recently, 300 EC patients with suspected gross cervical involvement that underwent hysterectomy between 1995 and 2009 were retrospectively analyzed having as primary endpoint the OS, and secondary endpoints the progression-free survival and adverse effects [35]. Seventy-four, 112, and 114 patients received RH, modified RH, and simple TH [35]. After a follow-up of 47 months, no significant difference among three type of hysterectomy was detected in any of the assessed endpoints, even if patients who received RH had longer operative time, higher rates of blood transfusion and severe urinary tract dysfunction [35].

Lymphadenectomy

The role of PEL and PAL in the treatment of EC at early stage is still debated.

Lymphadenectomy is highly important in determining a patient's prognosis and in tailoring adjuvant therapies [8]. However, two RCTs showed that PEL did not improve benefit in OS and DFS but it is associated with small statistically increase in perioperative complications and operative time [36,37]. May et al. [32], after data synthesis of the previous RCTs, confirmed the lack of significant difference in OS and DFS between women who received PEL and those who received no PEL (HR 1.07, 95%CI 081 to 1.43; and HR 1.23, 95%CI 0.96 to 1.58, respectively), but a risk significantly higher of systemic and local morbidity (RR 3.72, 95%CI 1.04 to 13.27, and RR 8.39, 95%CI 4.06 to 17.33, respectively) after nodes dissection. Although methodological limits were found in the two RCTs, it was evident that in early stage EC PEL should be delivered to the patients with clear indication.

Stage I EC patients present a lymph node metastasis in 10-12% of cases. Hence, many authors suggest a complete surgical staging for intermediate–high risk endometrioid cancer (stage IA G3 and IB) [8]. At this regard, at least 20 pelvic lymph nodes and at least 10 paraaortic lymph nodes up to the renal vessels should be removed. The incidence of isolated paraaortic lymph node metastasis in case of negative pelvic nodes is very low [38] but PAL should be always performed in high risk patients and/or in presence of pelvic metastasis at frozen section examination (about 50% of patients will have para-aortic metastasis) [39].

Regarding the PAL in early stage EC, no RCT has been designed to assess this issue. However, a recent wide retrospective cohort analysis study [40] on 671 EC patients demonstrated that a systematic lymphadenectomy (PEL plus PAL) in intermediate/high risk patients can improve the OS.

Several strategies have been employed to select patients with early stage EC for PEL/PAL.

Many surgeons tailor the PEL, and eventually the PAL, according to the myometrial infiltration assessed intra-operatively. To this regard, a recent meta-analysis [34] firstly confirmed the efficacy and the validity of intra-operative gross examination of myometrial invasion in patients with early stage EC. In addition, Chang et al. [33] demonstrated in a systematic review and meta-analysis the high diagnostic accuracy of FGD-PET/TC-PET to detect pelvic and/or para-aortic lymph nodes metastasis (up to 90% of cases) in untreated EC patients, suggesting a role to select patients to candidate to PEL and/or PAL. Contrarily, Kang et al. [41], in an other meta-analysis on 26 studies including 1101 procedures, sentinel lymph node biopsy showed a good diagnostic performance, even if definitive conclusion with impact on the clinical practice cannot be made for the small study effect.

Surgical Treatment

Surgical approaches to early stage EC include the traditional laparotomy; vaginal, laparoscopic and robotic assisted technique. In addition, several efforts have been made during the last years to reduce the invasiveness of the approach and several system and techniques have been employed in feasibility studies.

Furthermore, EC is diagnosed in women less than 40 years in 3-14% of all cases and >70% of them are nulliparous at the time of diagnosis [42]. In this set of patient, fertility sparing treatment is an essential topic to which it is possible to give some initial effective responses.

Laparotomy

Traditionally *laparotomic* approach has been considered the gold standard technique. In most cases a midline longitudinal laparotomy is performed that starts above the pubic symphysis and (depending on the extension of the lymphadenectomy) expands until the xiphoid.

Alternative ways of laparotomies are transverse incisions, such as the Pfannenstiel' or Cohen' incision, optionally with transection of the recti muscles (Maylard' incision) [43]. In some obese patients, laparotomy including a panniculectomy is performed [43].

With increasing body mass index (BMI), the rate of successful PEL/PAL is however significantly decreasing. The estimated blood loss rises and duration of surgery extends [44]. In morbidly obese patients noninfectious wound breakdown occurs in up to 10% [45].

Vaginal Surgery

This approach represents a safe alternative in high risk patient with limited operability and several morbidities. It is exclude the abdominal exploration and several abdominal procedures, i.e. PC, PEL/PAL, omentectomy, and so on.

A meta-analysis of RCTs on the risk/benefit ratio of the surgical approaches to hysterectomy for benign gynecological diseases concluded that the vaginal route should be, when feasible, always preferred [46]. In stage I EC patients, 5- and 10-year survival rates are 90% and 87%, respectively [47], similar findings were obtained also when bilateral adnexectomy was not performed [48]. This point can be crucial since up to 50% of the women treated with vaginal hysterectomy did not received adnexectomy in the clinical practice [48].

The vaginal approach can be employed in severely obese patients and in fragile patients, i.e. in elderly women or in women with co-morbidities limiting the general anesthesia, with a very low rate of surgical complications [49,50]. In these cases, the presence of risk factors of recurrence requiring a more extensive staging can drive a subsequent retroperitoneal staging by laparoscopy or a front-line radiotherapy [51].

Laparoscopic Surgery

In the last 15 years, the use of minimally invasive techniques has been widely accepted by many authors and it has been enclosed in European guideline as a feasible approach [8].

Actually, the feasibility, the safety and the efficacy of the laparoscopic approach for endometrial cancer has been clearly proven both in experimental and in clinical setting and both for stage I and stage II [52].

A recent meta-analysis of RCTs on a total of 8 studies, including 2310 patients treated with laparoscopy and 1389 treated with laparotomy, confirmed that the laparoscopic approach for surgical staging of early stage EC presents similar intraoperative complications but fewer postoperative complications than abdominal approach [53]. This difference translates in a significant cost-efficacy of laparoscopy over laparotomy [54]

That meta-analysis reported a laparoscopic conversion rate ranging between 0 and 25.8% [53]. This wide variation may be due to different preoperative selection criteria and heterogeneity in surgical skill [53] both in clinical trial than in clinical practice [52,55]. Several factors such as age, obesity, complexity of the surgical procedures, wide spread of disease, bleeding, heterogeneity in surgical skill and lack of standard criteria in performing laparoscopic hysterectomy cause wide variability in conversion rate.

In our experience, a very high conversion rate (about 50% of conversions) were due poor visualization of the operative field due to the impossibility to maintain the Trendelemburg's position for anesthesiology reasons [56]. To this regard, the amount of visceral fat, assessed by ultrasonography and/or computer tomography, rather than BMI, was identified as good predictor for conversion to laparotomy due to anesthesiology in obese patients with EC [57].

A recent paper suggested that an acceptable conversion rate should be less than 5% with a 70% of strategic and 30% of reactive conversion [58]. Generally, laparoscopy followed by an additional laparotomy is associated with substantially worse postoperative outcomes and prolonged hospital stay [58]. Moreover, our recent wide retrospective analysis [59] demonstrated that surgical and oncologic outcomes of converted patients are no different from those of patients staged successfully with laparoscopy or with laparotomy suggesting that the conversion to laparotomy should be not considered *per se* a complication. In fact, conversion should be considered a limit to the feasibility of the technique and it cannot be eliminated [60].

Nevertheless, actually every clinical early stage EC should be treated with laparoscopy approach. Several attempts has been made in literature to quantify the risk of conversion and to predict the probability of major adverse events [53], so to achieve the smaller conversion rate it is mandatory a full preoperatory evaluation of the risk factors but also to have a skilled and trained team.

To our knowledge, only one RCT [61] is available in literature aimed to assess surgical difference between laparoscopic-assisted vaginal hysterectomy (LAVH) and total laparoscopic hysterectomy (TLH). Even if almost all RCTs available used LAVH techniques, two surgical procedures revealed similar surgical outcome with a significant advantage in terms of shorter operating time in obese patients for TLH [61].

However, the laparoscopic approach to early stage EC is not only safe from a surgical point of view but also from an oncologic point of view. To this regard, Palomba et al. [62] showed no effect of the laparoscopy on OS (OR 0.96, 95%CI 0.51 to 1.81), DFS (OR 0.95, 95%CI 0.51 to 1.80), and cancer-related survival (OR 91; 95%CI 0.27 to 3.06). The lack of difference between laparoscopy and laparotomy for staging early stage EC has been also confirmed in the Gynecologic Oncology Group (GOG) LAP 2 study [63]. In particular, the difference between surgical approaches in recurrence rate at 3-year was of only 1.14 %.

Finally, a better quality of life (QoL) was observed in early stage EC patients who received laparoscopy when compared with those treated with laparotomy [5,64]. However, this benefit disappeared after 3 years from surgery [65]

Robotic Assisted Laparoscopic Surgery (RALS)

Robotic surgery introduced several improvements in the minimally invasive approach.

The advantages of robot assisted laparoscopic surgery (RALS) are the three-dimensional view; the possibility to wristed instruments such as laparotomy; the possibility to perform finer and delicate procedures because of robotic instruments provide improved dexterity and eliminate hand tremor; finally the decreasing in surgeon fatigue because of improved ergonomics [66]. Disadvantages are increased cost and operating time, lack of tactile feedback to the surgeon, additional surgical training required to become proficient on the system, large operating room size (secondary to the size of the robotic system), instrumentation limitations, and risk of mechanical failure intraoperatively [67].

When compared to laparotomy, total robotic hysterectomy (TRH) presented longer surgical time, but with a decrease in blood loss, transfusion rate, intra- and post-operative complications, and length of hospital stay [68,70]. When compared to standard laparoscopy, there was a consistent decrease in blood loss, although the true clinical impact of this is not clear. Indeed, in two of the largest studies directly comparing total laparoscopic hysterectomy (TLH) to TRH there was conflicting data about transfusion rate following surgery [69,70]. As for laparoscopy the rate of conversion to laparotomy was variable between studies.

Despite several studies have documented that lymph node yield is similar between robotic-assisted lymphadenectomy to traditional abdominal lymphadenectomy [62,63,68], it seems to be associated with a higher risk of lymphedema than laparotomy [71,72].

The rate of lymphedema after PEL for gynecologic malignancies varies widely in the literature (1–37%) and is most often underreported. The risk of developing lymphedema may increase with the number of lymph nodes removed [73,74]. a recent study from Japan noticed a significant increase in lymphedema with removal of the lymph nodes distal to the deep circumflex iliac vein [74]. The improved visibility and exposure may result in resection of deeper lymph nodes in the obturator space and around the deep circumflex iliac vein. Since the circumflex iliac nodes are rarely positive in grade 1 endometrioid adenocarcinomas leaving these nodes in place should be considered [75].

TRH and TLH show similar intra- and post-operative complication rates and types of complications. As with TLH, the rate of complications is significantly decreased when comparing TRH to TAH [69]. Moreover, several studies show a significant decrease in conversion rate when a TRH is performed compared to TLH [69,70]. Because the most common cause of conversion in TLH is, as already stated, the poor visualization of the operating field, this limit is overcome by robotic surgery [70].

Another cause of conversion from laparoscopy to laparotomy is the high BMI, which is a common findings in EC patients; the conversion rate of TRH to TAH is lower than that of TLH with comparable BMI. Robotic surgery might be indicated in this group of patients to reduce the rate of conversion [76,77]. However it should be taken in mind that TRH takes longer time, and obese patients have less efficient ventilation [78] during pneumoperitoneum. This risk should be compared with the benefit of an early hospital discharge [77].

As for TLH, complications of the vaginal cuff, such as leakage of peritoneal fluid and cuff dehiscence, are a common concern for patients undergoing TRH [79,80]. The rate of vaginal cuff complications reported in literature is of 1–4% [81,82]. Cuff dehiscence may be related to the use of electrosurgical instrumentation to incise or open the vagina which may compromise blood supply and healing [81]. Other potential risk factors for cuff dehiscence include the magnification afforded by the robotic platform which may result in incorporation of less vaginal epithelium in the cuff closure, as well as the potential for excessive tension used to tie knots [81]. Also an early return to physical activity may lead to increased abdominal and vaginal pressure. Usually cuff dehiscence is diagnosed between three and six weeks. Suture methods varied among surgeons to include running and interrupted polyglycolic acid sutures. However this concern is still debated.

Because TRH seems to present similar morbidity but increased cost compared with TLH, some authors suggest to wait for comparative long-term efficacy data before to justify its widespread use [76].

Laparoendoscopic Single-Site Surgery (LESS)

Preliminary results suggested an early postoperative benefit in terms of postoperative pain for the laparoendoscopic single-site surgery (LESS) patients compared to standard LPS patients [83-85].

Some authors used the same surgical technique of the LESS approach as for standard TLH because single access surgery should be like the standard laparoscopic technique in order to maintain safety, reproducibility, and oncologic criteria [83]. Specific limitations of single-port surgery, such as reduced visualization, loss of triangulation, and instrument interference, was reported by Ramirez [86]. Some technical solutions [87] were proposed to perform a total LESS hysterectomy (LESSH) without an additional port [88]: 1. use of a 5-mm 30 telescope with a flexible handle or alternatively, a 5-mm video laparoscope with a flexible tip; 2. use of two straight instruments of different lengths (43 and 33 cm long) or double-bent instruments to reduce clashing and changing; 3. multifunctional instruments that are able to grasp, coagulate, and dissect; 4. uterine manipulator reducing the limits due to the absence of an auxiliary port; and 5. closure of the uterine artery at the origin, after adequate extraperitoneal dissection and ureter visualization, to reduce the need of bipolar coagulation at the paracervical region, with lower risk of bleeding and ureter injury.

Recently Escobar reported the technique and the feasibility of single-port laparoscopic pelvic and para-aortic node sampling and lymphadenectomy [89].

Probably, progressive improvement in surgical skills, could facilitate the use of the total LESSH procedure by decreasing the initial difficulties related to this new approach by progressively lowering the operative time and offering some advantages in terms of less invasiveness, faster recovery time, less postoperative pain, and better cosmetic outcome.

A recent study evaluated the feasibility and the safety of robotic single-site hysterectomy (RSSH) in low risk early EC. Seventeen procedures were performed and only one conversion to standard vaginal surgery was necessary because of a BMI of 52 kg/m^2, the result of problems of hypercapnia [90].

Single-site robotic surgery has the advantages of LESS, including improved cosmetic result and less postoperative pain, but the automatic reversion of the crossed instruments allows far greater maneuverability and ergonomics than other LESS methods [87]. It also provides an improved three-dimensional image, and the semirigid, curved instrumentation offers a stable and safe platform with lack of instrument collisions [91].

Moreover, this system allows a rotation of the camera and of the instruments of about 45° in both sides, facilitating the execution of the surgical procedure. Single-site port procedures require a specific training of the team because before proceeding with insertion, one must verify that the port is clamped correctly. Incorrect clamping of the port may cause difficulties during the operation, especially when the port is partly torn or damaged. Also, cannula placement and the docking process, although not difficult, require additional training of the team. A certain limitation of the Single-Site platform is that the semiflexible robotic instruments are not yet articulated (as in multiport robotic surgery), which means that there are fewer degrees of freedom compared to multiport robotic surgery. The cannulae are rather long, which determines a quite small distance between the instrument and uterus. This makes the technique harder than single-port laparoscopy. Another disadvantage of this platform is the lack of a bipolar coagulation device and monopolar scissors, which would be useful during bleeding near critical structures and for the lymphadenectomy [90].

Recently, the first case-control study compared RSSH with LESSH for early EC. Few not clinically relevant differences were registered so the two approaches resulted comparable, in terms of operative time, blood loss and conversion/complication rate [92].

As for robotic surgery in generally, this procedure is aggravated by high direct and indirect costs, the real benefit of RSSH respect the LESSH and multiport robotic surgery it is still debated.

Mini/Micro Laparoscopy

The mini and microlaparoscopy are two minimally invasive approaches consisting in the use of access ports smaller in comparison with those used for traditional laparoscopic approach in order to reduce the incision-related morbidity and to minimize the stress response to surgery. These procedure are also commonly called "needlescopic" surgery because after surgery there are only very small skin scars.

Commonly, the term "minilaparoscopy" refers to the use of a central 5-mm abdominal access for laparoscope and 3-mm ancillary ports, whereas "microlaparoscopy" to the use of 3-mm laparoscopic access for laparoscope and 2-mm ancillary ports. These procedure were initially employed for diagnostic procedures or minor therapeutic manoeuvres (adhesions lysis, tubar sterilization, ovarian drilling, second-look laparoscopies).

The first procedures were performed in the 90s by Gagner et al. [93]. However, these surgical techniques did not became popular because the instruments are deemed by several surgeons too fragile and, then, expensive.

Ghezzi et al. [94] published the first series of TH performed using minilparoscopic approach and demonstrated an high feasibility of the procedure also for major gynecological surgery. Further studies [95] assessed the feasibility and the safety of the "needlescopic surgery" also for staging early stage EC. Of note, EC patients were staged with TH and SO and PEL, whereas PAL was omitted. No difference was detected in comparison with historical controls in any of the parameters assessed, whereas less postoperative pain and a reduce hospital stay was recorded in EC patients who underwent microlaparoscopic staging [95].

Recently, a RCT compared the minilaparoscopic approach versus LESS to perform TH even in patients not specifically selected for EC [96] . That study demonstrated a significant advantage of mini-laparoscopy over the LESS in terms of operative time and postoperative pain suggesting the potential best efficacy of the minilaparoscopic surgery also in early stage EC who need TH and SO.

Natural Orifice Translumental Endoscopic Surgery (NOTES) and Minilaparoscopic-Assisted Natural Orifice Surgery (MANOS)

Natural orifice translumental endoscopic surgery (NOTES) is a term coined by a multidisciplinary consortium of gastroenterologists and surgeons in order to define "scarless" surgical techniques.

The first description of NOTES was of Kalloo et al. in 2004 [97]. The researchers performed a peritoneoscopy and liver biopsy though transgastric approach [97]. Only one year later, there was the first gynecological procedure for tubal ligation in a porcine model [98].

For gynecological surgery and, specially, for gynecological oncology the clinical application of NOTES was not progressing, neither in animal and human model, for the lack of development of specific flexible endoscopes. In consideration of the long learning curve for this new instrumentations and equipments, it is possible in the next future the application of robotic surgery to these platforms.

However, in the recent years it is common practice to use hybrid NOTES, such as the transvaginal route for the extraction of surgical specimens. This is the case of the extraction of lymph nodes in endobag through vagina during mini/micro-laparoscopic laparoscopy. The term commonly used is "minilaparoscopic-assisted natural orifice surgery (MANOS)" techniques which include all surgical procedures characterized by the use of natural orifices for some surgical gestures with the support from mini-laparoscopy and not necessarily the use of flexible instrumentation [99].

Mixed Laparoscopic Techniques

Two Port Access (TPA) Laparoscopy

The TPA system consisted of a single multichannel port at the umbilicus and an ancillary 5-mm port in the suprapubic area [100-102]. Lee et al. [100] evaluated the feasibility and safety of TPA laparoscopy in gynecologic oncology. Eighty-one consecutive patients (29 early stage EC patients) who underwent TPA laparoscopic surgery for various gynecologic cancers were analyzed in a retrospective fashion. All surgical procedures were completed laparoscopically with no conversion to laparotomy, and in only 2 cases 1 or 2 additional ports were required. The rate of complication was lower than 5% [101].

The same group of researchers compared longitudinally surgical outcomes of TPA laparoscopy with the conventional one in early stage EC patients [102]. Surgical data of 21 subjects who received TPA laparoscopy were compared with those from 42 age- and BMI-matched patients who underwent conventional staging laparoscopy in the same period. No conversion was detected in both groups. TPA group had a significantly longer operating time, more paraaortic nodes retrieved, shorter postoperative hospital stay, and less postoperative pain.

Isobaric/Gasless Laparoscopy

As above underlined, a proportion of EC patients, especially if obese, are converted to laparotomy for anesthesiologic concerns due to Trendelenburg position. In addition, traditional laparoscopy is performed under general anesthesia and its use is limited by several pathophysiologic changes induced by pneumoperitoneum, such as reduction of pulmonary function, increased dead space, increased pulmonary wedge pressure, effect on cardiac output and increase in arterial carbon dioxide tension [103-106]. To this regard, pneumoperitoneum is contraindicated in patients with impaired cardiopulmonary function and clinical practice guidelines from the European Association for Endoscopic Surgery recommend that all patients should be preoperatively assessed for the presence of cardiac comorbidities [105,106].

Recently, a new subcutaneous lifting system to perform laparoscopy (Laparotenser®; Lucini Surgical Concepts, Milan, Italy), has been experimented representing a relatively new technique with several potential advantages for both patient and surgeon. It is characterized by 2 curved pluriplan needles with blunt tips that, introduced subcutaneously through 2 pubic skin incisions of 2 mm each and suspended from a mechanical arm attached to a rigid pillar, lift the abdominal wall for an optimal pelvic exposure.

Primary access is generally achieved by the insertion of a 10-mm trocar through a intraumbilical or sovraumbelical incision, whereas further accesses are performed according to surgeon' preference under direct visualization. Specifically, it is possible also to perform a skin incision of 4 cm in order to permit the use the conventional instrumentation and surgical technique.

A recent prospective analysis on a little sample of 15 EC patients seems to suggest the efficacy and safety of the Laparotenser® for treating gynecological malignancies, and its usefulness in case of patients at high-risk for cardio-vascular complication [107].

Specific Complication of the Minimally Invasive Laparoscopic Approaches: The Port-Site Metastases (PMS)

Specific complications of minimally invasive laparoscopic approaches include: vaginal cuff recurrences and port-site metastases (PSMs).

Vaginal cuff recurrence is a rare complication of the laparoscopic procedures. Several Authors have related this complication with the length of the resected vagina and with the uterine manipulator use. However, controlled data seem to reassure about the efficacy of the length of vagina excised by laparoscopy [108] and the use of uterine manipulator on the surgical outcome in EC patients [109]

PSMs are an uncommon complication reported to occur in 1–2% of all laparoscopic procedures for gynecological malignancies, which is similar to rates of wound metastases following open surgery [110]. Currently, there is growing interest in PSM after minimally invasive treatment of gynecological cancers. This interest is probably due to the increasing use of laparoscopy and robotic surgery in gynecologic oncology, particularly in EC.

The real incidence of PSMs after surgery for EC remains uncertain but it is probably underreported. Using a broader definition than Reymond's standard criteria [111], PSMs consists in cancer recurrence in the scar tissue at 1 or more trocar sites or at the incision wound after laparoscopy without peritoneal carcinosis. It's clear that it is always need a careful evaluation of concurrent and occult metastases with the use of invasive (i.e., diagnostic laparoscopy) or noninvasive (i.e., positron emission tomography) methods, even if this last option is expensive and unable to detect microscopic metastases.

At the moment, 6 cases of PSM have been reported in early stage EC treated with both conventional laparoscopy or RALS [110,112,113]. In only one case, the PSM were "non isolated" [114].

In case of PSM, the risk that this metastasis is related to peritoneal carcinosis is at least double that found in the absence of peritoneal disease ("true" or "isolated" PSM). Actually, risk factors for PSMs are not well identified, it could be related to the stage and histology. Non-isolated PSMs were diagnosed in the 90% of cases in advanced-stage EC, whereas an aggressive histologic condition and a high grade were found, respectively, in 50% and 60% of the subjects. Conversely, in 75% of the patients with isolated PSMs, EC in early stages were diagnosed at the first surgery [110].

In early stage EC, intraoperative complications might favor dissemination of neoplastic cells such as difficult uterine extraction caused by uterine leiomyomata, uterine perforation [111] and micro-trauma of the tissues. Finally, malignancy contamination did not appear to be related to direct contact with cancer tissues. In fact, in a high proportion of cases, PSMs were not found at the extraction ports or at the wider ports.

The same doubts exist on the preventive measures, several and different strategies were adopted among studies: trocar site irrigation, suture of the fascia and of the peritoneum, use of an extraction bag, tubal coagulation , deflation with the port in place, low intra-abdominal pressure, use of vagina for the extraction bag, and no uterine manipulation [110]. The inclusion of the laparoscopic ports in the radiotherapy fields could be also suggested in patients requiring external beam radiotherapy [110,111].

However, no prophylactic strategy can be considered to show proven efficacy because of the lack of data regarding the impact of PSMs with respect to different strategies [110].

Also the treatment of PSMs is debated. Non-isolated PSMs should be treated with chemotherapy. The management of isolated PSMs is more complex. PSM should be managed with a wide excision of the lesion, frozen section evaluation, and if the metastasis is confirmed, a diagnostic laparoscopy with peritoneal washing and peritoneal biopsies should be performed to exclude occult metastases. If other sites of recurrence are carefully excluded, local radiotherapy can be an adequate treatment.

Both patients with ''non-isolated'' and ''isolated'' PSMs present a poor prognosis, and it is questionable whether PSM, although defined as ''isolated,'' could be really considered an ''isolated'' disease or whether it could be the expression of a hidden, disseminated, micrometastatic disease representing the "tip of an iceberg" [56].

Fertility Sparing Surgery

A progressive delay in the age of first conception has been seen in Western countries over the last few decades, resulting in an increased frequency of nulliparous in the young EC patient population and in the increasing of the papers about fertility sparing treatment.

Several are the attempts published about the fertility-sparing treatment for early stage EC patients regard essentially hormonal treatments, whereas very little has been published on the fertility-sparing surgery [115].

Actually there is no consensus on the best way to preserve fertility in young early stage EC patients. Recently, the main criteria for admitting a woman to a fertility-sparing program were clarified. They include deep motivation to preserve fertility, EC type 1 with grade 1 lesions, and no myometrial invasion or extrauterine spread evaluated with magnetic resonance imaging and/or laparoscopy. Nevertheless, in a low percentage of cases, even in grade 1 EC there is a risk of pelvic (3%) and paraaortic (1.7%) lymph node involvement, deep myometrial invasion (9%), spread of tumor to the adnexa (6%), and coexisting ovarian neoplasms (19%). Moreover, fertility-sparing treatment of grade 1 EC is associated with a risk of disease progression of 5%-6% [115]. Thus, patients should be counseled regarding these additional risks.

Recently, local surgical resection combined to hormonal therapy has been successfully experimented [116].

However, hormonal management is the best consolidated treatment for young women with early stage EC desiring childbearing [117-121]. Finally, the use of ovulation induction drugs after conservative treatment of EC did not increase the recurrence of the disease [122,123]. Moreover, resulting pregnancy seemed to have an advantageous effect on the oncologic outcome [122].

On the basis of available data of the literature, all the fertility sparing treatments should be considered as experimental therapies. All patients should be followed-up as long as pregnancy is desired, and until the end of childbearing age. Successively, standard radical surgery should be performed.

Conclusion

In a high proportion of cases EC is diagnosed in early stage. The optimal treatment and staging for early stage EC is still controversial, even if the extra fascial TH plus salpingo-oophorectomy seems to be the crucial surgical procedures influencing the OS and the DFS. Thus, several minimally invasive approaches have been developed and experimented for early stage EC.

The traditional laparoscopy should be considered the gold standard in these cases since it combines the mini-invasiveness to the possibility of an extensive staging that include also PC evaluation, and PEL and/or PAL.

If possible, the robotic assistance can help the surgeon. In obese EC patients with comorbidity vaginal or isobaric gasless laparoscopy under loco-regional anesthesia can be an option.

Even if to be considered experimental, all new surgical approaches could give similar results of the traditional laparoscopy in expert and skilled hands reducing further the surgical trauma. Moreover, the preference of a specific surgery should not never influence the choice for an adequate oncologic staging if needed.

References

[1] Bakkum-Gamez JN, Gonzalez-Bosquet J, Laack NN, Mariani A, Dowdy SC. Current issues in the management of endometrial cancer. *Mayo Clin Proc* 2008;83:97-112.

[2] Ferlay J, Shin HR, Bray F, Forman D, Mathers C, Parkin DM. Estimates of worldwide burden of cancer in 2008: GLOBOCAN 2008. *Int J Cancer* 2010;127:2893-917.

[3] Amant F, Moerman P, Neven P, Timmerman D, Van Limbergen E, Vergote I. Endometrial cancer. *Lancet* 2005;366:491-505.

[4] Bray F, Loos AH, Oostindier M, Weiderpass E. Geographic and temporal variations in cancer of the corpus uteri: incidence and mortality in pre- and postmenopausal women in Europe. *Int J Cancer* 2005;117:123-31.

[5] Janda M, Gebski V, Brand A, Hogg R, Jobling TW, Land R, et al. Quality of life after total laparoscopic hysterectomy versus total abdominal hysterectomy for stage I endometrial cancer (LACE): a randomised trial. *Lancet Oncol* 2010;11:772-80.

[6] Pecorelli S. Revised FIGO staging for carcinoma of the vulva, cervix, and endometrium. *Int J Gynaecol Obstet* 2009;105:103-4.

[7] Mandato VD, Formisano D, Pirillo D, Ciarlini G, Cerami LB, Ventura A, et al. Province wide clinical governance network for clinical audit for quality improvement in endometrial cancer management. *Int J Gynecol Cancer* 2012;22:94-100.

[8] Colombo N, Preti E, Landoni F, Carinelli S, Colombo A, Marini C, et al., ESMO Guidelines Working Group. Endometrial cancer: ESMO Clinical Practice Guidelines for diagnosis, treatment and follow-up. *Annals of Oncology* 2011;22:35-9.

[9] Creutzberg CL, van Putten WL, Koper PC, Lybeert ML, Jobsen JJ, Wárlám-Rodenhuis CC, et al. Surgery and postoperative radiotherapy versus surgery alone for patients with stage 1 endometrial carcinoma: multi centre trial. PORTEC study group. *Lancet* 2000;355:1404-11.

[10] Keys HM, Roberts JA, Brunetto VL, Zaino RJ, Spirtos NM, Bloss JD, et al.; Gynecologic Oncology Group: A phase III trial of surgery with or without adjunctive external pelvic radiation therapy in intermediate risk endometrial adenocarcinoma: a Gynecologic Oncology Group study. *Gynecol Oncol* 2004;92:744-51.

[11] ASTEC/EN.5 Study Group, Blake P, Swart AM, Orton J, Kitchener H, Whelan T, Lukka H, et al. Adjuvant external beam radiotherapy in the treatment of endometrial cancer (MRC ASTEC and NCIC CTG EN.5 randomised trials): pooled trial results, systematic review, and meta-analysis. *Lancet* 2009;373:137-46.

[12] Furukawa N, Takekuma M, Takahashi N, Hirashima Y. Intraoperative Evaluation of Myometrial Invasion and Histological Type and Grade in Endometrial Cancer: Diagnostic Value of Frozen Section. *Archives of Gynecology and Obstetrics* 2010;281:913-7.

[13] Pristauz G,. Bader A, Regitnig P, Haas J, Winter R, Tamussino K. How Accurate is Frozen Section Histology of Pelvic Lymph Nodes in Patients with Endometrial Cancer? *Gynecologic Oncology* 2009;115:12-7.

[14] Creasman WT, Morrow CP, Bundy BN, Homesley HD, Graham JE, Heller PB. Surgical pathologic spread patterns of endometrial cancer. A Gynecologic Oncology Group Study. *Cancer* 1987;60:2035-41.

[15] Lurain JR, Rumsey NK, Schink JC, Wallemark CB, Chmiel JS. Prognostic significance of positive peritoneal cytology in clinical stage I adenocarcinoma of the endometrium. *Obstet Gynecol* 1989;74:175-9.

[16] Harouny VR, Sutton GP, Clark SA, Geisler HE, Stehman FB, Ehrlich CE. The importance of peritoneal cytology in endometrial carcinoma. *Obstet Gynecol* 1988;72:394-8.

[17] Hirai Y, Fujimoto I, Yamauchi K, Hasumi K, Masubuchi K, Sano Y. Peritoneal fluid cytology and prognosis in patients with endometrial carcinoma. *Obstet Gynecol* 1989;73:335-8.

[18] Lurain JR. The significance of positive peritoneal cytology in endometrial cancer. *Gynecol Oncol* 1992;46:143-4.

[19] Takeshima N, Nishida H, Tabata T, Hirai Y, Hasumi K. Positive peritoneal cytology in endometrial cancer: enhancement of other prognostic indicators. *Gynecol Oncol* 2001;82:470-3.

[20] Kadar N, Homesley HD, Malfetano JH. Positive peritoneal cytology is an adverse factor in endometrial carcinoma only if there is other evidence of extrauterine disease. *Gynecol Oncol* 1992;46:145-9.

[21] Morrow CP, Bundy BN, Kurman RJ, Creasman WT, Heller P, Homesley HD, et al. Relationship between surgical-pathological risk

factors and outcome in clinical stage I and II carcinoma of the endometrium: a Gynecologic Oncology Group study. *Gynecol Oncol* 1991;40:55-65.

[22] Zaino RJ, Kurman RJ, Diana KL, Morrow CP. Pathologic models to predict outcome for women with endometrial adenocarcinoma: the importance of the distinction between surgical stage and clinical stage--a Gynecologic Oncology Group study. *Cancer* 1996;77:1115-21.

[23] Milosevic MF, Dembo AJ, Thomas GM. The clinical significance of malignant peritoneal cytology in stage I endometrial carcinoma. *Int J Gynecol Cancer* 1992;2:225-35.

[24] Grimshaw RN, Tupper WC, Fraser RC, Tompkins MG, Jeffrey JF. Prognostic value of peritoneal cytology in endometrial carcinoma. *Gynecol Oncol* 1990;36:97-100.

[25] Kasamatsu T, Onda T, Katsumata N, Sawada M, Yamada T, Tsunematsu R, et al. Prognostic significance of positive peritoneal cytology in endometrial carcinoma confined to the uterus. *Br J Cancer* 2003;88:245-50.

[26] Tebeu PM, Popowski Y, Verkooijen HM, Bouchardy C, Ludicke F, Usel M, et al. Positive peritoneal cytology in early-stage endometrial cancer does not influence prognosis. *Br J Cancer* 2004;91:720-4.

[27] Havrilesky LJ, Cragun JM, Calingaert B, Alvarez Secord A, Valea FA, et al. The prognostic significance of positive peritoneal cytology and adnexal/serosal metastasis in stage IIIA endometrial cancer. *Gynecol Oncol* 2007;104:401-5.

[28] Saga Y, Imai M, Jobo T, Kuramoto H, Takahashi K, Konno R, Ohwada M, Suzuki M. Is peritoneal cytology a prognostic factor of endometrial cancer confined to the uterus? *Gynecol Oncol* 2006;103:277-80.

[29] Orezzoli JP, Sioletic S, Olawaiye A, Oliva E, del Carmen MG. Stage II endometrioid adenocarcinoma of the endometrium: clinical implications of cervical stromal invasion. *Gynecol Oncol* 2009;113:316-23.

[30] Wright JD, Fiorelli J, Kansler AL, Burke WM, Schiff PB, Cohen CJ, et al. Optimizing the management of stage II endometrial cancer: the role of radical hysterectomy and radiation. *Am J Obstet Gynecol* 2009;200:419.e1-7.

[31] Signorelli M, Lissoni AA, Cormio G, Katsaros D, Pellegrino A, Selvaggi L, et al. Modified radical hysterectomy versus extrafascial hysterectomy in the treatment of stage I endometrial cancer: results from the ILIADE randomized study. *Ann Surg Oncol* 2009;16:3431-41.

[32] May K, Bryant A, Dickinson HO, Kehoe S, Morrison J. Lymphadenectomy for the management of endometrial cancer. *Cochrane Database Syst Rev* 2010;CD007585.

[33] Chang MC, Chen JH, Liang JA, Yang KT, Cheng KY, Kao CH. 18F-FDG PET or PET/CT for detection of metastatic lymph nodes in patients with endometrial cancer: a systematic review and meta-analysis. *Eur J Radiol* 2012;81:3511-7.

[34] Mavromatis ID, Antonopoulos CN, Matsoukis IL, Frangos CC, Skalkidou A, Creatsas G, et al. Validity of intraoperative gross examination of myometrial invasion in patients with endometrial cancer: a meta-analysis. *Acta Obstet Gynecol Scand* 2012;91:779-93.

[35] Takano M, Ochi H, Takei Y, Miyamoto M, Hasumi Y, Kaneta Y, et al. Surgery for endometrial cancers with suspected cervical involvement: is radical hysterectomy needed (a GOTIC study)? *Br J Cancer* 2013;109:1760-5

[36] Benedetti Panici P, Basile S, Maneschi F, Alberto Lissoni A, Signorelli M, et al. Systematic pelvic lymphadenectomy vs. no lymphadenectomy in early-stage endometrial carcinoma: randomized clinical trial. *J Natl Cancer Inst* 2008;100:1707-16.

[37] ASTEC study group. Efficacy of systematic pelvic lymphadenectomy in endometrial cancer (MRC ASTEC trial): a randomised study. *Lancet* 2009; 373:125-36.

[38] Boronow RC. Endometrial Cancer and Lymph Node Surgery: The Spins Continue - A Case for Reason. Gynecologic Oncology 2008;111:3-6.

[39] Delpech Y, Barranger E. Management of Lymph Nodes in Endometrioid Uterine Cancer. *Current Opinion in Oncology* 2010;22:487-91.

[40] Todo Y, Kato H, Kaneuchi M, Watari H, Takeda M, Sakuragi N. Survival effect of para-aortic lymphadenectomy in endometrial cancer (SEPAL study): a retrospective cohort analysis. *Lancet* 2010;375:1165-72.

[41] Kang S, Yoo HJ, Hwang JH, Lim MC, Seo SS, Park SY. Sentinel lymph node biopsy in endometrial cancer: meta-analysis of 26 studies. *Gynecol Oncol* 2011;123:522-7.

[42] Signorelli M, Caspani G, Bonazzi C, Chiappa V, Perego P, Mangioni C. Fertility-sparing treatment in young women with endometrial cancer or atypical complex hyperplasia: a prospective single-institution experience of 21 cases. *BJOG* 2009;116:114-8.

[43] Fagotti A, Ferrandina G, Longo R, Mancuso S, Scambia G. Minilaparotomy in Early Stage Endometrial Cancer: An Alternative to

Standard and Laparoscopic Treatment. *Gynecologic Oncology* 2002;86:177-83.

[44] Foley K, Lee RB. Surgical Complications of Obese Patients with Endometrial Carcinoma. *Gynecologic Oncology* 1990;39:171-4.

[45] Pavelka JC, Ben-Shachar I, Fowler JM, Ramirez NC, Copeland LJ, Eaton LA, et al. Morbid Obesity and Endometrial Cancer: Surgical, Clinical and Pathologic Outcomes in Surgically Managed Patients. *Gynecologic Oncology* 2004;95:588-92.

[46] Nieboer TE, Johnson N, Lethaby A, Tavender E, Curr E, Garry R, et al. Surgical approach to hysterectomy for benign gynaecological disease. *Cochrane Database Syst Rev* 2009:CD003677.

[47] Massi G, Savino L, Susini T. Vaginal hysterectomy versus abdominal hysterectomy for the treatment of stage I endometrial adenocarcinoma. *Am J Obstet Gynecol* 1996;174:1320-6.

[48] Chan JK, Lin YG, Monk BJ, Tewari K, Bloss JD, Berman ML. Vaginal Hysterectomy as Primary Treatment of Endometrial Cancer in Medically Compromised Women. *Obstet Gynecol* 2001;97:707-11.

[49] Susini T, Massi G, Amunni G, Carriero C, Marchionni M, Taddei G, Scarselli G. Vaginal hysterectomy and abdominal hysterectomy for treatment of endometrial cancer in the elderly. *Gynecol Oncol* 2005;96:362-7.

[50] Smith SM, Hoffman MS. The role of vaginal hysterectomy in the treatment of endometrial cancer. *Am J Obstet Gynecol* 2007;197:202.e1-6; discussion 202.e6-7.

[51] Dowdy SC, Aletti G, Cliby WA, Podratz KC, Mariani A. Extra-peritoneal Laparoscopic Para-aortic Lymphadenectomy-A Prospective Cohort Study of 293 Patients with Endometrial Cancer. *Obstet Gynecol* 2008;111:418-24.

[52] Palomba S, Ghezzi F, Falbo A, Mandato VD, Annunziata G, Lucia E, et al. Laparoscopic versus abdominal approach to endometrial cancer: a 10-year retrospective multicenter analysis. *Int J Gynecol Cancer* 2012;22:425-33.

[53] Zullo F, Falbo A, Palomba S. Safety of laparoscopy vs laparotomy in the surgical staging of endometrial cancer: a systematic review and metaanalysis of randomized controlled trials. *Am J Obstet Gynecol* 2012;207:94-100.

[54] Bijen CB, Vermeulen KM, Mourits MJ, Arts HJ, Ter Brugge HG, van der Sijde R, et al. Cost effectiveness of laparoscopy versus laparotomy

in early stage endometrial cancer: a randomised trial. *Gynecol Oncol* 2011;121:76-82.

[55] Fanning J, Hossler C. Laparoscopic conversion rate for uterine cancer surgical staging. *Obstet Gynecol* 2010;6:135-57.

[56] Palomba S, Mandato VD, La Sala GB. Isolated port-site metastasis after robotic hysterectomy for stage IA endometrial adenocarcinoma. *Obstet Gynecol* 2014;123:664.

[57] Palomba S, Nelaj E, Zullo F. Visceral fat amount as predictive factor for early laparotomic conversion in obese patients with endometrial cancer. *Gynecol Oncol* 2006;102:128-9.

[58] Twijnstra AR, Blikkendaal MD, van Zwet EW, Jansen FW. Clinical relevance of conversion rate and its evaluation in laparoscopic hysterectomy. *J Minim Invasive Gynecol* 2013;20:64-72.

[59] Palomba S, Ghezzi F, Falbo A, Mandato VD, Annunziata G, Lucia E, et al. Conversion in endometrial cancer patients scheduled for laparoscopic staging: a large multicenter analysis. *Surg Endosc* 2014 (andrebbe aggiornato ma non so se è in press o meno).

[60] Yang C,Wexner SD, Safar B, et al. Conversion in laparoscopic surgery: does intraoperative complication influence outcome? *Surg Endosc* 2009;23:2454-8.

[61] Ghezzi F, Cromi A, Bergamini V, Uccella S, Beretta P, Franchi M, Bolis P. Laparoscopic-assisted vaginal hysterectomy versus total laparoscopic hysterectomy for the management of endometrial cancer: a randomized clinical trial. *J Minim Invasive Gynecol* 2006;13:114-20.

[62] Palomba S, Falbo A, Zullo F. Updating of a recent meta-analysis of randomized controlled trials to assess the safety and the efficacy of the laparoscopic surgery for treating ealy stage endometrial cancer. *Gynecol Oncol* 2009;114:135-6.

[63] Walker JL, Piedmonte MR, Spirtos NM, Eisenkop SM, Schlaerth JB, Mannel RS, et al. Recurrence and survival after random assignment to laparoscopy versus laparotomy for comprehensive surgical staging of uterine cancer: Gynecologic Oncology Group LAP2 Study. *J Clin Oncol* 2012;30:695-700.

[64] Zullo F, Palomba S, Russo T, Falbo A, Costantino M, Tolino A, et al. A prospective randomized comparison between laparoscopic and laparotomic approaches in women with early stage endometrial cancer: a focus on the quality of life. *Am J Obstet Gynecol* 2005;193:1344-52.

[65] Zullo F, Palomba S, Falbo A, Russo T, Mocciaro R, Tartaglia E, et al. Laparoscopic surgery vs laparotomy for early stage endometrial cancer:

long-term data of a randomized controlled trial. *Am J Obstet Gynecol* 2009;200:296.e1-9.
[66] Satava RM. Robotic surgery: From past to future-A personal journey. *Surg Clin North Am* 2003;83:1491.
[67] Tinelli A, Malvasi A, Gustapane S, Buscarini M, Gill IS, Stark M, et al. Robotic assisted surgery in gynecology: current insights and future perspectives. *Recent Pat Biotechnol* 2011;5:12-24.
[68] DeNardis SA, Holloway RW, Bigsby GE 4th, Pikaart DP, Ahmad S, Finkler NJ. Robotically assisted laparoscopic hysterectomy versus total abdominal hysterectomy and lymphadenectomy for endometrial cancer. *Gynecol Oncol* 2008;111:412-7.
[69] Boggess JF, Gehrig PA, Cantrell L, Shafer A, Ridgway M, Skinner EN, et al. A comparative study of 3 surgical methods for hysterectomy with staging for endometrial cancer: Robotic assistance, laparoscopy, laparotomy. *Am J Obstet Gynecol* 2008;199:360 e1-360 e9.
[70] Seamon LG, Cohn DE, Henretta MS, Kim KH, Carlson MJ, Phillips GS, et al. Minimally invasive comprehensive surgical staging for endometrial cancer: Robotics or laparoscopy? *Gynecol Oncol* 2009;113:36-41.
[71] Barnett JC, Havrilesky LJ, Bondurant AE, Fleming ND, Lee PS, Secord AA, et al. Adverse events associated with laparoscopy vs laparotomy in the treatment of endometrial cancer. *Am J Obstet Gynecol* 2011;205:1-6.
[72] Ackes FJ, Brudie LA, Farrell MR, Ahmad S, Finkler NJ, Bigsby GE, et al. Short- and long-term morbidity and outcomes after robotic surgery for comprehensive endometrial cancer staging. *Gynecol Oncol* 2012;125:546-51.
[73] Abu-Rustum NR, Alektiar K, Iasonos A, Lev G, Sonoda Y, Aghajanian C, et al. The incidence of symptomatic lower-extremity lymphedema following treatment of uterine corpus malignancies: a 12-year experience at Memorial Sloan-Kettering Cancer Center. *Gynecol Oncol* 2006;103:714–8.
[74] Todo Y, Yamamoto R, Minobe S, Suzuki Y, Takeshi U, Nakatani M, et al. Risk factors for postoperative lower-extremity lymphedema in endometrial cancer survivors who had treatment including lymphadenectomy. *Gynecol Oncol* 2010;119:60-4.
[75] Todo Y, Kato H, Okamoto K, Minobe S, Suzuki Y, Ohba Y, et al. Incidence of metastasis in circumflex iliac nodes distal to the external iliac nodes in intermediate and high-risk endometrial cancer. Gynecol Oncol 2011;122:55-8.

[76] Wright JD, Burke WM, Wilde ET, Lewin SN, Charles AS, Kim JH, et al. Comparative effectiveness of robotic versus laparoscopic hysterectomy for endometrial cancer. *J Clin Oncol* 2012;30:783-91.

[77] Lowery WJ, Leath CA 3rd, Robinson RD. Robotic surgery applications in the management of gynecologic malignancies. *J Surg Oncol* 2012;105:481-7.

[78] Sprung J, Whalley DG, Falcone T, Warner DO, Hubmayr RD, Hammel J. The impact of morbid obesity, pneumoperitoneum, and posture on respiratory system mechanics and oxygenation during laparoscopy. *Anesth Analg* 2002;94:1345-50.

[79] Robinson BL, Liao JB, Adams SF, Randall TC. Vaginal cuff dehiscence after robotic total laparoscopic hysterectomy. *Obstet Gynecol* 2009;114:369-71.

[80] Kho RM, Akl MN, Cornella JL Magtibay PM, Wechter ME, Magrina JF. Incidence and characteristics of patients with vaginal cuff dehiscence after robotic procedures. *Obstet Gynecol* 2009;114:231-5.

[81] Cronin B, Sung VW, Matteson KA. Vaginal cuff dehiscence: risk factors and management. *Am J Obstet Gynecol* 2012;206:284-8.

[82] Uccella S, Ghezzi F, Mariani A, et al. Vaginal cuff closure after minimally invasive hysterectomy: our experience and systematic review of the literature. *Am J Obstet Gynecol* 2011;205:119.e1-12.

[83] Fagotti A, Rossitto C, Marocco F, Gallotta V, Bottoni C, Scambia G, et al. Perioperative outcomes of laparoendoscopic single-site surgery (LESS) versus conventional laparoscopy for adnexal disease: a case-control study. *Surg Innov* 2011;18:29-33.

[84] Yim GW, Jung YW, Paek J. Transumbilical single-port access versus conventional total laparoscopic hysterectomy: surgical outcomes. *Am J Obstet Gynecol* 2010;203:26.e1-26.e6.

[85] Kim TJ, Lee YY, Cha HH. Single-port-access laparoscopic- assisted vaginal hysterectomy versus conventional laparoscopic-assisted vaginal hysterectomy: a comparison of perioperative outcomes. *Surg Endosc* 2010;24:2248-52.

[86] Ramirez PT. Single-port laparoscopic surgery. Is a single incision the next frontier in minimally invasive gynecologic surgery? Gynecol Oncol 2009;114:143-4.

[87] Fanfani F, Rossitto C, Gagliardi ML, Gallotta V, Gueli Alletti S, Scambia G, et al. Total laparoendoscopic single-site surgery (LESS) hysterectomy in low-risk early endometrial cancer: a pilot study. *Surg Endosc* 2012;26:41-6.

[88] Lee YY, Kim TJ, Kim CJ. Single-port access laparoscopicassisted vaginal hysterectomy: a novel method with a wound retractor and a glove. *J Minim Invasive Gynecol* 2009;16:450-3.

[89] Escobar PF, Fader AN, Rasol N. Single-port laparoscopic pelvic and para-aortic node sampling or lymphadenectomy: development of a technique and instrumentation. *Int J Gynecol Cancer* 2010;20:1268-73.

[90] Vizza E, Corrado G, Mancini E, Baiocco E, Patrizi L, Fabrizi L, et al. Robotic single-site hysterectomy in low risk endometrial cancer: a pilot study. *Ann Surg Oncol* 2013;20:2759-64.

[91] Escobar PF, Fader AN, Paraiso MF, Kaouk JH, Falcone T. Robotic-assisted laparoendoscopic single-site surgery in gynecology: initial report and technique. *J Minim Invasive Gynecol* 2009;16:589-91.

[92] Fagotti A, Corrado G, Fanfani F, Mancini M, Paglia A, Vizzielli G, et al. Robotic single-site hysterectomy (RSS-H) vs. laparoendoscopic single-site hysterectomy (LESS-H) in early endometrial cancer: a double-institution case-control study. *Gynecol Oncol* 2013;130:219-23.

[93] Gagner M, Garcia-Ruiz A. Technical aspects of minimally invasive abdominal surgery performer with needlescopic instruments. *Surg Laparosc Endosc* 1998;8:171-9.

[94] Ghezzi F, Cromi A, Siesto G, Boni L, Uccella S, Bergamini V, et al. Needlescopic hysterectomy: incorporation of 3-mm instruments in total laparoscopic hysterectomy. *Surg Endosc* 2008;22:2153-7.

[95] Ghezzi F, Cromi A, Siesto G, Zefiro F, Franchi M, Bolis P. Microlaparoscopy: a further development of minimally invasive surgery for endometrial cancer staging -- initial experience. *Gynecol Oncol* 2009;113:170-5.

[96] Fanfani F, Fagotti A, Gagliardi ML, Monterossi G, Rossitto C, Costantini B, et al. Minilaparoscopic versus single-port total hysterectomy: a randomized controller study. *J Minim Invasive Gynecol* 2013;20:192-7.

[97] Kalloo AN, Singh VK, Jagannath SB, Niiyama H, Hill SL, Vaughn CA, et al. Flexible transgastric peritoneoscopy: a novel approach to diagnostic and therapeutic interventions in the peritoneal cavity. *Gastrointest Endosc* 2004;60:114-7.

[98] Jagannath SB, Kantsevoy SV, Vaughn CA, Chung SS, Cotton PB, Gostout CJ, et al. Peroral transgastric endoscopic ligation of fallopian tubes with long-term survival in porcine model. *Gastrointest Endosc* 2005;61:449-53.

[99] Noguere JF, Cuadrado A. NOTES, MANOS, SILS and other new laparoendoscopic techniques. *W J Gastrointest Endosc* 2012;4:212-7.

[100] Lee M, Nam EJ, Kim S, Kim JH, Kim YT, Kim SW. Two-port access laparoscopic surgery in gynecologic oncology. *Int J Gynecol Cancer* 2013;23:935-42

[101] Paek J, Nam EJ, Jung YW, Lee SH, Kim JH, Kim YT, et al. Two-port access staging laparoscopy for gynecologic cancers: a pilot study. J Laparoendosc *Adv Surg Tech A* 2010;20:347-53.

[102] Paek J, Nam EJ, Lee M, Yim GW, Kim S, Kim YT, et al. Two-port access versus conventional staging laparoscopy for endometrial cancer. *Int J Gynecol Cancer* 2012;22:515-20.

[103] Marret H, Chevillot M, Giraudeau B. Study Group of the French Society of Gynaecology and Obstetrics (Ouest Division). Factors influencing laparoconversions during the learning curve of laparoscopic myomectomy. *Acta Obstet Gynecol Scand* 2006;85:324-9.

[104] O'Malley C, Cunningham AJ. Physiologic changes during laparoscopy. *Anesthesiol Clin North America* 2001;19:1-19.

[105] Neudecker J, Sauerland S, Neugebauer E, Bergamaschi R, Bonjer HJ, Cuschieri A, et al. The European Association for Endoscopic Surgery clinical practice guideline on the pneumoperitoneum for laparoscopic surgery. *Surg Endosc* 2002;16:1121-43.

[106] Palomba S, Zupi E, Falbo A, Russo T, Marconi D, Zullo F. New tool (Laparotenser) for gasless laparoscopic myomectomy: a multicenter-controlled study. *Fertil Steril* 2010;94:1090-6.

[107] Pellegrino A, Damiani GR, Tartagni M, Speciale D, Villa M, Sportelli C, et al. Isobaric laparoscopy using LaparoTenser system in surgical gynecologic oncology. *J Minim Invasive Gynecol* 2013;20:686-90.

[108] Palomba S, Falbo A, Zullo F. Reply: Observations on the role of assisted laparoscopic surgery in patients with early stage endometrial cancer. *Am J Obstet Gynecol* 2010;202:e20; author reply e20-1.

[109] Lee M, Kim YT, Kim SW, Kim S, Nam EJ. Effects of uterine manipulation on surgical outcomes in laparoscopic management of endometrial cancer: a prospective randomized clinical trial. *Int J Gynecol Cancer* 2013;23:372-9.

[110] Palomba S, Falbo A, Russo T, La Sala GB. Port-site metastasis after laparoscopic surgical staging of endometrial cancer: a systematic review of the published and unpublished data. *J Minim Invasive Gynecol* 2012;19:531-7.

[111] Reymond MA, Schneider C, Kastl S, Hohenberger W, Köckerling F. The pathogenesis of port-site recurrences. *J Gastrointest Surg* 1998;2:406-14.

[112] Lonnerfors C, Bossmar T, Persson J. Port-site metastases following robotic-assisted laparoscopic surgery for gynecological malignancies. *Acta Obstet Gynecol Scand* 2013 (in press).

[113] Grabosh S, Xynos F. Isolated port-site metastasis after robotic hysterectomy for stage I endometrial adenocarcinoma. *Obstet Gynecol* 2013;122:437-9.

[114] Palomba S, Falbo A, Oppedisano R, Russo T, Zullo F. Isolated port-site metastasis after laparoscopic surgery for endometrial cancer: a case report. *Gynecol Oncol Rep* 2012;2:16-7.

[115] Martinez A, Poilblanc M, Ferron G, De Cuypere M, Jouve E, Querleu D. Fertility-preserving surgical procedures, techniques. *Best Pract Res Clin Obstet Gynaecol* 2012;26:407-24.

[116] Mazzon I, Corrado G, Masciullo V, Morricone D, Ferrandina G, Scambia G. Conservative surgical management of stage IA endometrial carcinoma for fertility preservation. *Fertil Steril* 2010;93:1286-9.

[117] Signorelli M, Caspani G, Bonazzi C, Chiappa V, Perego P, Mangioni C. Fertility-sparing treatment in young women with endometrial cancer or atypical complex hyperplasia: a prospective single-institution experience of 21 cases. *BJOG* 2009;116:114-8.

[118] Minig L, Franchi D, Boveri S, Casadio C, Bocciolone L, Sideri M. Progestin intrauterine device and GnRH analogue for uterus-sparing treatment of endometrial precancers and well-differentiated early endometrial carcinoma in young women. *Ann Oncol* 2011;22:643-9.

[119] Nucera G, Mandato VD, Gelli MC, Palomba S, La Sala GB. Gonadotropin releasing hormone agonist and levonorgestrel-intrauterine device followed by in vitro fertilization program as management strategy for an infertile endometrial cancer patient: a case report. *Gynecol Endocrinol* 2013;29:219-21.

[120] Chiva de Agustín L, Lapuente Sastre F, Corraliza Galán V, Granados Galainena L, González Martín A, González Cortijo L, et al. Conservative management of patients with early endometrial carcinoma: a systematic review. *Clin Transl Oncol* 2008;10:155-62.

[121] Gunderson CC, Fader AN, Carson KA, Bristow RE. Oncologic and reproductive outcomes with progestin therapy in women with endometrial hyperplasia and grade 1 adenocarcinoma: a systematic review. *Gynecol Oncol* 2012;125:477-82.

[122] Ichinose M, Fujimoto A, Osuga Y, Minaguchi T, Kawana K, Yano T, et al. The influence of infertility treatment on the prognosis of endometrial cancer and atypical complexendometrial hyperplasia. *Int J Gynecol Cancer* 2013;23:288-93.

[123] Park JY, Seong SJ, Kim TJ, Kim JW, Kim SM, Bae DS, Nam JH. Pregnancy outcomes after fertility-sparing management in young women with early endometrial cancer. *Obstet Gynecol* 2013;121:136-42.

In: Endometrial Cancer
Editors: I. Diaz-Padilla, J. Garcia-Donas
ISBN: 978-1-63321-323-4

Chapter VI

Radiation Therapy in Early-Stage Endometrial Cancer

Millie Light[1] and Melanie Powell[2]
[1]University College Hospital, London, UK
[2]St Bartholomew's Hospital, London, UK

Abstract

Adjuvant treatment for uterine cancer is now defined according to risk of recurrence. Although radiotherapy has not been shown to confer a survival benefit for women with uterine cancer it does improve loco-regional control. This chapter summarises and discusses by risk group the recent data for adjuvant radiation in endometrial cancer.

Introduction

The use of radiation therapy to treat endometrial cancer has a long history dating back to first reports in 1909. Early therapies involved treatment such as radium packing and Heyman (1935) reported a 58.2% 5-year survival for early stage patients using the 'Stockholm' method. Initial use of radiotherapy techniques was in the pre-operative setting but by the 1980's this was on the decline and moved towards delivery almost exclusively in the post- operative, adjuvant setting.

In modern day practice the role of post operative radiotherapy for early stage disease has become a topic of controversy and while the majority of cases are successfully treated with surgery alone, those with risk factors associated with poorer prognosis can hope for a reduction in local and regional recurrence with adjuvant treatment but studies have suggested no overall survival benefit.

Staging and Prognostic factors

The majority of endometrial tumours are of epithelial origin commonly endometrioid adenocarcinoma accounting for 75% of cases [1]. Non-endometrioid histological types are associated with a poorer prognosis and include serous, mucinous and clear cell with around 3% of all tumours demonstrating sarcomatous pathology [2] Prognosis in endometrial cancer is also related to stage and the presence of several other pathological risk factors such as depth of myometrial invasion, lymphovascular space invasion, tumour grade and volume and cervical involvement.

The FIGO 2010 (International Federation of Gynaecology and Obstetrics) staging system reflects the pattern of local and distant spread of the disease, including lymph node spread. Over 80% of newly diagnosed endometrial cancers are confined to the uterus (FIGO Stage 1-2) and considered early stage with a good prognosis and overall survival of around 85-90% [1]. More advanced disease with regional involvement has lower survival rates of 60-65% [6].

Patterns of disease spread may be local extension along the endometrial surface to eventually include the lower segment, cervix and parametria, or a more infiltrating pattern may see the disease invade the depth of the endometrium to extend into the myometrium, serosa and peritoneal cavity and lymphatic spread.

In the absence of other distant diseases, lymph node metastasis is the most significant prognostic factor [3]. Once the sub-serosa is breached, lymphatic invasion is common and subsequent lymph node involvement is higher. The first echelon nodes are typically the internal and external iliac chain although isolated para-aortic involvement can be found in some 1-3.5% of cases [3,4]. Even the earliest stage cancers, however, can show unexpected lymph node involvement. Between 0-7% of Stage 1A and 17-25% of Stage 1B have pelvic or para-aortic lymph node involvement [4]. This is more likely with higher grade tumours and where lymphovascular space invasion is present. Less than 1% of stage 1A grade 1 tumours had nodal disease.

Haematogenous spread is less frequent in endometrial cancers and tends to occur late in the disease. The most common sites of metastases include the lungs, liver and bones.

Risk Stratification for Early Disease

A recent analysis of SEER (Surveillance, Epidemiology and End Result) data suggests survival is increased in early stage, lower grade disease and in younger women [5]. Broadly, disease can be considered as early (Stage 1-2), locally advanced (Stage 3-4A) or metastatic (stage 4B) based on this staging scheme. As the drive to further improve outcomes looks to identify higher risk cases, adjuvant therapy and management is often based on further stratifying this group of early stage disease based on the presence of other risk factors (table 1) which can point towards low, intermediate and high risk of recurrence.

Adjuvant Radiation Therapy in Early Disease

Low Risk, FIGO (2010) Stage 1A Grade 1-2

Most retrospective studies suggest a favourable outcome for early disease (stage 1, grade 1-2 disease) when treated with surgery alone. Prospective studies detailed below come to the consensus that those without high risk factors have a low risk of loco-regional relapse and treatment in this group may lead to additional treatment related deaths with increased morbidity and recommend adjuvant therapy is omitted. In a large prospective study, the GOG reported a 5-yr survival rate of 92.7% for surgical stage 1 patients with no other adverse features other than Grade and myometrial invasion [11]. In reviewing data from these prospective trials it is important to appreciate the changes in the FIGO staging system from 1988-2010 and the stage migration with some cases of low risk disease being upstaged to reflect changes in prognosis.

Table 1. Risk recurrence based on Pathology

RISK	PATHOLOGY
LOW RISK	Stage 1a grade 1 / 2
INTERMEDIATE RISK	Stage IA grade 3, Stage 1A with LVSI, Stage IB grade 1/2, Stage II grade 1/2
HIGH RISK	Stage IA (invasion) G3 with LVSI, Stage IB grade 3, Any Stage II Any serous or clear cell

Intermediate Risk Disease, FIGO (2010) Stage 1B-2 Grade 1-2, or Stage 1A with Either G3 or LVSI

Four prospective randomised trials (GOG-99 1987-95[11]. The Norwegian Aalders trial 1968-75[12], PORTEC 1990-97[13], and ASTEC/EN5 1996-2005[14]) evaluated the role of post-operative pelvic irradiation in intermediate risk groups. The FIGO 1988 staging system is used within these studies.

PORTEC 1

This study aimed to define whether adjuvant pelvic radiotherapy improved both locoregional control and survival for women with stage I endometrial cancer. Eligibility was based on pathological stage with inclusion criteria being: grade I with deep myometrial invasion, grade 2 with any invasion and grade 3 with superficial invasion.

Following hysterectomy, 715 patients were randomised to pelvic irradiation or no further treatment and no vaginal brachytherapy was given. Pelvic radiotherapy reduced locoregional recurrence (4 vs 14%) but there was no survival benefit. The majority of patients with locoregional failure were successfully salvaged, with 3-year survival of 75% for those with isolated vaginal recurrence compared to 69 and 13% for patients with pelvic or distant relapse. Multivariate analysis showed age greater than 60 to be a risk factor for a poorer outcome for both local control (4 vs 10%) and death from endometrial cancer (4 vs 9%). As might be expected, long-term complications were higher in the radiotherapy group (25 vs 6%), however, significant complications were rare with only 2% of grade 3 or 4.

GOG-99 Trial

This trial looked at the addition of external beam radiotherapy and involved 448 women with surgically staged (lymphadenectomy included) 'intermediate-risk' early endometrial cancer. Following surgery randomisation was either to whole pelvic radiation or observation. At two years there was a reduced incidence of locoregional recurrence in the treatment arm (3 vs 12%, $p = 0.0007$) but there was no significant improvement in survival with radiation. The 4-year estimated survival was 86% in the control arm and 92% in the radiation arm ($p = 0.557$). A sub group analysis was carried out on a 'high intermediate risk' (HIR) group based on age, in addition to deep myometrial invasion, grade and LVSI. In GOG 99, women younger than 50 years had to have all 3 histologic risk factors to be considered HIR, but if they were 50-70 years they were considered HIR if they had 2 histologic risk factors and HIR if over 70 and 1 risk factor. The benefit of radiotherapy was highest in this HIR group with a two year incidence of recurrence of 26 vs 6%.

MRC ASTEC Study

This was an international study set up by the Medical Research Council (UK) with two trials within one; a surgical and an adjuvant radiotherapy study. The radiotherapy trial was designed to evaluate the role of pelvic radiotherapy in women with early stage disease and pathological features suggestive of intermediate- or high-risk of recurrence. The similar Canadian National Cancer Institute EN.5 study started at the same time but when it was realised that insufficient numbers were being accrued to complete this trial the MRC invited the CNIC in 1998 to combine their data with ASTEC. A total of 905 patients (789 ASTEC, 116 EN.5) were randomised following surgery to either pelvic radiotherapy or no external beam radiotherapy. In ASTEC, brachytherapy was permitted in either group if it was a centre's standard policy and in EN.5 brachytherapy was given according to local policy. The 5-year overall survival was identical in both groups at 84%. There was a small benefit in terms of isolated local recurrence 6% in the observation group versus 3% in the radiotherapy group. This, however, includes a very small number of women since only one third (42 of 120) recurrences were isolated to the pelvis. It should be noted that, 53% of all participants received brachytherapy, and, purely by chance, the proportion was similar in each arm with 51% in the observation group and 53% in the pelvic radiotherapy group. As would be anticipated, toxicity was greater in women receiving external beam radiotherapy. Acute toxicity was 27% in the observation group versus 57% in the pelvic radiotherapy group. Late toxicity was seen in 45 and 61% of the observation and external beam groups with severe problems in 3 and 8% respectively.

PORTEC 2

Due to the concerns about potential toxicity of external beam pelvic radiotherapy, the role of vaginal brachytherapy alone in uterine-confined disease has been evaluated in PORTEC 2, the follow on trial of PORTEC 1. It developed from the findings of PORTEC 1 that showed patients in the high intermediate-risk group have improved local control with the addition of radiotherapy (5 versus 19% local recurrence) with 75% of recurrences occurring in the vagina. With a treatment related complication rate of 25% and phase 2 data suggesting vault brachytherapy was as effective at reducing the incidence of vaginal recurrence as external beam treatment, the phase 3 PORTEC 2 trial was devised. It aimed to answer the question of whether vaginal vault brachytherapy is sufficient treatment to prevent vaginal recurrence. Patients falling into the high intermediate-risk group with the following features were included in the study; age greater than 60 and FIGO 1998 stage IC (outer third invasion) grade 1 or 2, or stage IB (middle third invasion) grade 3, stage IIA (except grade 3 extending into the outer half of the myometrium). Over 400 patients were randomised to either external beam radiotherapy or vaginal vault brachytherapy. At three years the vaginal and pelvic recurrence rates were similar at 2 and 3.5% in the brachytherapy arm versus 1 and 0.6% in the external beam arm. Distant relapse rates were 5.7% with external beam versus 6.3% with brachytherapy. Additionally brachytherapy led to reduced toxicity and better quality of life.

Conclusions from these trials and meta-analysis looking at pelvic radiotherapy in stage 1 endometrial cancer suggest a higher significant improvement in local control is conferred, but with no clearly demonstrated survival advantage[7]. GOG found an increase in local control and progression free survival but no overall survival advantage however, these trials were underpowered for high risk cases and both PORTEC-1 and PORTEC-2 specifically excluded patients with 1998 FIGO stage 1C (outer third myometrial invasion), grade 3 endometrial carcinoma (FIGO stage IB, grade 3), thus the use of adjuvant brachytherapy alone in the highest risk subset remains undetermined.

High Risk Stage I-2A Disease

The number of patients with Stage 1 grade 3, deep myometrial invasion is low in the studies mentioned and therefore firm data is lacking. In view of the higher rates of local and distant recurrence found at subgroup analysis these patients may be offered external beam radiotherapy with or without vaginal vault brachytherapy. Two large retrospective SEER analyses [15,16] and a subset review of the meta-analyses of the prospective trials[17], suggests there might possibly be a survival advantage in using radiotherapy in these high risk groups. The question remains as to whether or not survival is compromised due to extra-pelvic metastatic disease and whether effective systemic adjuvant chemotherapy in addition to radiotherapy should be used. To resolve this issue an intergroup trial of the Dutch Cooperative Gynaecologic Oncology Group has conducted the PORTEC 3 study, a randomized trial comparing concurrent chemoradiation and adjuvant chemotherapy with pelvic radiation alone in high-risk and advanced-stage endometrial carcinoma (Stage IA (invasion) plus grade 3 and LVSI; stage IB or II grade 3; stage III; stage I A (invasion), B, II or III with serous or clear cell pathology).

Unfavourable Histological Subtypes

Similarly those with unfavourable histological subtypes, uterine serous and clear cell, have an increased incidence of extra-uterine disease and lower 5-year survival rates than endometrioid carcinoma. The EORTC 55991 and PORTEC 3 studies included these patients to assess the role of chemotherapy in addition to radiotherapy and the full results are awaited leaving external beam radiotherapy as a suitable adjuvant therapy at present.

Summary

The role of adjuvant radiotherapy in endometrial cancer has become a contentious issue. For low-risk stage I disease no adjuvant treatment is necessary and for intermediate- risk vaginal vault brachytherapy is probably adequate. However, in high-risk early cancer and advanced disease the optimal management is far from clear. Although pelvic radiotherapy improves locoregional control it does not improve survival. Therefore in women who have undergone hysterectomy and pelvic lymphadenectomy its role continues to be questioned. The role of adjuvant chemotherapy in this high-risk group remains very pertinent and the Dutch led international PORTEC 3 which closed at the end of 2013 may well produce results which clarify the adjuvant treatment of this group of patients.

References

[1] Creasman, WT; Odicino, F; Maisonneuve; et al. Carcinoma of the corpus uteri. FIGO 26th Annual report on the results of treatment in Gynaecological cancer. *Iny J. Gynaecol Obstet*, 2006, 95, Suppl 1, S105-143

[2] Christopherson, WM; Connelly, PJ; Alberhasky, RC; et al. Carcinoma of the endometrium: V. An analysis of prognosticators in patients with favorable subtypes and stage I disease. *Cancer*, 1983; 51: 1705-1709

[3] Creasman, WT; Morrow, CP; Bundy, BN; et al. Surgical pathologic spread patterns of endometrial cancer. A Gynecologic Oncology Group Study. *Cancer*, 1987, 60, 2035-2041

[4] Morrow, CP; Bundy, BN; Kurman, RJ; et al. Relationship between surgical-pathological risk factors and outcome in clinical stage I and II carcinoma of the endometrium. A Gynecologic Oncology Group study. *Gynecol Oncol*, 1991, 40, 55-65

[5] Chan, JK; Sherman, AE; Kapps, DS; et al. Influence of gynaecologic oncologists on the survival of patients with endometrial cancer. *J Clin Oncol*, 2011, 29, 832-838

[6] Alketruse, SF; Kosary, CL; Krapcho, M. *SEER cancer statistics review.* Bethesda MD: National Cancer Institute, 1975-2007.

[7] Kong, A; Simera, I; Collingwood, M; Williams, C; Kitchener, H. on behalf of Cochrane Gynaecological Cancer Group. Adjuvant radiotherapy for stage I endometrial cancer: systematic review and meta-analysis. *Ann Oncol*, 2007, 18, 1595-1604 & updated Cochrane database systematic review 2012-01-02

[8] Soliman, PT; Frumovitz, M; Spannuth, W; et al. Lymphadenectomy during endometrial cancer staging: practice patterns among gynaecologic oncologists. *Gynaecol Oncol*, 2010, 119, 291-294

[9] Havrilesky, LJ; Cragun, JM; Calingaert, B; et al. resection of lymph node metastases influences survival in Stage IIIc endometrial cancer. *Gynaecol Oncol*, 2005, 99, 689-695.

[10] Todo, Y; Kato, H; Kaneuchi, M; et al. Survival effect of para-aortic lymphadenectomy in endometrial cancer (SEPAL study): a retrospective cohort analysis. *Lancet*, 2010, 375, 1165-1172.

[11] Keys, HM; Roberts, JA; Brunetto, VL; et al. A phase III trial of surgery with or without adjunctive external pelvic radiation therapy in intermediate risk endometrial adenocarcinoma: a Gynaecologic Oncology Group study. *Gynaecol Oncol*, 2004, 92, 744-751

[12] Aalders, J; Abeler, V; Kolstad, P; Onsrud, M. Postoperative external irradiation and prognostic parameters in stage I endometrial carcinoma:clinical and histopathologic study of 540 patients: *Obstet Gynecol*, 1980, 56, 419-427.

[13] Creutzberg, CL; van Putten, WL; Koper, PC; et al. Surgery and postoperative radiotherapy versus surgery alone for patients with stage-1 endometrial carcinoma: multicentre randomised trial. PORTEC Study Group. Post Operative Radiation Therapy in Endometrial Carcinoma. *Lancet*, 2000, 355, 1404-1411.

[14] Blake, P; Swart, AM; Orton, J; et al. Adjuvant external beam radiotherapy in the treatment of endometrial cancer (MRC ASTEC and NCIC CTG EN.5 randomised trials): pooled trial results, systematic review, and meta-analysis. *Lancet*, 2009, 373, 137-146.

[15] Chino, JP; Jones, E; Berchuck, A; et al. The influence of Radiation Modality and Lymph Node Dissection on Survival in Early Stage Endometrial cancer. *Int J Radia Oncol Biol Phys*, 2011.

[16] Lee, CM; Szabo, A; Shrieve, DC; et al. Frequency and effect of adjuvant radiation therapy among women with stage 1 endometrial adenocarcinoma. *JAMA*, 2006, 295, 389-97.

[17] Onsrud, M; Cvancarova, M; Hellebust, TP; et al. Long-term outcomes after pelvic radiation for early-stage endometrial cancer. *J Clin Oncol*, 2013, 31, 3951-3956.

In: Endometrial Cancer
Editors: I. Diaz-Padilla, J. Garcia-Donas
ISBN: 978-1-63321-323-4

Chapter VII

The Role of Adjuvant Chemotherapy in Endometrial Cancer

Thomas Hogberg*
Department of Cancer Epidemiology, University of Lund,
University Hospital, Lund, Sweden

Summary

Adjuvant radiotherapy, either external beam radiotherapy or vaginal brachytherapy, can effectively eradicate micrometastases within the irradiated field but have no impact on overall survival. Hence, when an endometrial cancer has metastasized locally, it has frequently also implanted distant metastases. Adjuvant therapy should therefore include systemic treatment. Chemotherapy, mainly with platinum compounds, taxanes, and anthracyclines render high response rates in advanced or recurrent endometrial cancer, but this translates in only modest improvements in progression-free and overall survival. Better systemic treatments need to be developed. The knowledge about the molecular mechanisms driving endometrial cancer is expanding and possible targets for therapy have been identified. The combination of

* Corresponding author: Email: thomas.hogberg@med.lu.se.

radiotherapy and chemotherapy appears promising as adjuvant therapy in early high-risk endometrial cancer. Ongoing randomized clinical trials will hopefully soon resolve pending questions about the role of different treatment modalities in the adjuvant therapy of endometrial cancer

Introduction

Endometrial cancer (EC) is the most common gynecologic cancer in the western world. It is estimated that worldwide almost 300,000 women were diagnosed with EC and 75,000 died of the disease in 2008 [1]. EC mainly affects postmenopausal women with a median age between 65-70 years. Many patients have concurrent comorbidities, such as obesity, diabetes, and cardiovascular diseases. The incidence (age-standardized to the United States population 2000) in the US is 27 per 10^5 womenyears [2]. The Nordic Cancer Registries estimated that despite unchanged age-standardized incidence over the next 2 decades the absolute number of cases will increase by 20% because of the ageing and the increasing obesity of the population [3]. EC generally has a good prognosis due to early diagnosis, with 75% of patients having stage I disease, but per stage the survival is about the same as for ovarian cancer [4, 5]. Advanced EC had even worse outcome than ovarian cancer in a case-control study [6]. As reported in the FIGO (International Federation of Gynecology and Obstetrics) Annual Report [4] there is a substantial variation in survival rates among patients with stage I EC, with subgroups having high risk for micrometastatic disease (e.g. FIGO 2009 stage IB grade 3). Bokhman proposed the concept of type I and type II endometrial carcinomas based on clinical behavior and histopathology [7]. Type I being good prognosis estrogen related tumors of the endometrioid type stemming from a background of endometrial hyperplasia and type II non-estrogen related mainly non-endometrioid (e.g. serous and clear cell) carcinomas with worse prognosis arising from a background of atrophic endometrium. Modern molecular biology has further supported this classification [8, 9].

Pelvic external beam radiotherapy (EBRT) has been the traditional adjuvant therapy. Randomized studies comparing adjuvant EBRT with observation have failed to show an improvement in OS despite that around 70% of progressions within the irradiated field were prevented [10]. Thus, most patients with local micro-metastatic disease also have dissemination outside the irradiated field and there is a need for systemic adjuvant therapy, either added to, or instead of radiotherapy. Recently even the role for radiation in advanced disease has been questioned [11].

Risk Groups

The vast majority of patients are primarily treated with surgery (total hysterectomy and bilateral salpingo-oophorectomy). Major prognostic factors for EC predicting metastatic disease are stage, age, histological type, grade, depth of myometrial invasion and presence of lymph-vascular space invasion (LVSI). Pelvic and para-aortic lymphadenectomy, if performed, informs about microscopic lymph-node dissemination [12, 13].

Risk groups for stage I EC in the 2009 FIGO staging system [14]:

- **Low risk**: Stage IA grade 1-2 and endometrioid type EC
- **Intermediate risk**: Stage IA grade 3 or IB grades 1-2 and endometrioid type EC
- **High intermediate risk**: Age of at least 60 years and/or LVSI and Stage IA grade 3 or IB grades 1-2 and endometrioid type EC
- **High risk**: IB grade 3 endometrioid type EC or stage II-III or non-endometrioid types of EC.

The majority of patients with EC have low to intermediate (55%) or high-intermediate (30%) risk features, while only 15% have a high-risk profile. Five-year survival rates for patients with intermediate risk EC are 80-85%. Most of these patients die of intercurrent diseases; the rate of endometrial cancer death is 8-10%.

Chemotherapy

Phase 2 studies on chemotherapy (CT) in advanced or metastatic endometrial cancer have shown response rates exceeding 20% mainly with anthracyclines, platinum compounds, and taxanes [15, 16]. Two randomized studies compared doxorubicin and cisplatin (AP) with doxorubicin (A) [17, 18]. Both studies found that the combination gave better response rates but no significant differences in survival. AP was for many years regarded as the standard CT in endometrial cancer (Table 1).

Table 1. Selected phase II and III chemotherapy studies in advanced or recurrent endometrial cancer

Reference	Type of trial	Intervention	n	Study population	ORR %	mPFS months	mOS months
Aapro 2003 (17)	Phase-III	Doxorubicin Doxorubicin+cisplatin	87 90	Chemonaive	17 43	7 8	7 9
Thigpen 2004 (18)	Phase-III	Doxorubicin Doxorubicin+cisplatin	150 131	Chemonaive	25 42	4 6	9 9
Fleming 2004 (25)	Phase-III	Doxorubicin+cisplatin Doxorubicin+cisplatin+paclitaxel	129 134	Chemonaive	34 57	5 8	12 15
Hoskins 2001 (26)	Phase-II	Paclitaxel-carboplatin	63	Mixed	61	n.r.	n.r.
Sorbe 2008 (27)	Phase-II	Paclitaxel-carboplatin	66	Mixed	67	14	26
Akram 2005 (28)	Retrospective Phase-II	Paclitaxel-carboplatin	18	Chemonaive	63	24	27
Michener 2005 (29)	Retrospective Phase-II	Paclitaxel-carboplatin	22	Mixed	87	n.r	n.r.
Scudder 2005 (30)	Phase-II	Paclitaxel-carboplatin	47	Chemonaive	40	7	14
Arimoto 2007 (31)	Phase-II	Paclitaxel-carboplatin	37	Mixed population	61	n.r	n.r.
Muggia 2002 (19)	Phase-II	Liposomal doxorubicin	42	Pretreated	8.5	n.r.	8.2
Homesley 2005 (20)	Phase-II	Liposomal doxorubicin	52	Chemonaive	12	n.r.	11
Balbi 2007 (21)	Phase II	Liposomal doxorubicin	22	Chemonaive	36	n.r.	n.r.
Pignata 2007 (24)	Phase-II	Liposomal doxorubicin+carboplatin	42	Chemonaive	60	12	18
Vandenput 2009 (38)	Phase II	Paclitaxel+carboplatin	30	Chemonaive	74	13	23

mOS: Median overall survival, mPFS: Median progression-free survival, n: Number of patients, n.r.: Not reported, ORR: Overall response rate.

Phase-II results regarding liposomal doxorubicin as single drug in endometrial cancer have been contradictory. GOG discarded liposomal doxorubicin as an interesting drug in endometrial cancer [19, 20], while Balbi and colleagues [21] found a 36% response rate. The combination of liposomal doxorubicin and carboplatin has shown equal activity as paclitaxel and carboplatin and (TcP) in ovarian cancer [22]. In recurrent or advanced endometrial cancer, two fairly large phase 2 trials found response rates of 44% and 52% with a favorable toxicity profile [23, 24].

The Gynecology Oncology Group (GOG) tested the addition of paclitaxel (T) to AP in 273 (263 eligible) women with advanced or metastatic endometrial cancer of any cell type [25]. Response rate (57% vs 34%), PFS (median 8.3 vs 5.3 months) and OS (median 15.3 vs 12.3 months) were significantly better with TAP. However, the TAP combination was toxic—the rate of grade 2–3 peripheral neurotoxicity was 39% compared with 5% in the AP arm. All women in the TAP arm received a granulocyte stimulator (filgrastim). The imbalance in the number of possibly treatment-related deaths (five on TAP vs none on AP) is of note. However, only two of the five deaths (neutropenic fever and AML) were, according to the authors, clearly treatment-related. The modest gains and the reservations about the toxicity of this regimen have precluded widespread use.

Paclitaxel and carboplatin (TcP) is a commonly used well-tolerated drug combination in gynecologic cancer. However, neurotoxicity is still problematic. Phase 2 studies and retrospective studies in endometrial cancer have demonstrated high response rates (40%–90%) [26-31]. The Japanese Gynecologic Oncology Group (JGOG) compared the efficacy and safety of the different combinations of taxanes and platinum agents, i.e., TcP, docetaxel + cisplatin (DP), docetaxel + carboplatin (DcP), and paclitaxel + cisplatin (TP) in JGOG-2041, a phase II randomized study [32]. TP was eliminated, as the results of clinical trials for ovarian cancer had revealed a strong neurotoxicity compared with TcP. The response rates of the three regimens were not inferior to AP therapy and the toxicity was acceptable. The response rate to DcT (48%) was somewhat, although not significantly, lower than to TcP (60%) and DP (52%). TcP and DP were therefore selected for comparison with AP in a randomized phase III trial, JGOG-2043. Advanced cases with residual tumors no greater than 2 cm, and patients with stage I and II with invasion to more than half of the myometrium and histological grade 2 or 3 of all cell types were eligible. JGOG-2043 has closed but the final results have not yet been reported [33].

The large randomized GOG-209 trial compared TAP with TcP in patients with advanced FIGO stage III or IV or recurrent EC of all cell types. Results of GOG-209 were presented at the Society of Gynecologic Oncologist´s Annual Meeting on Women´s Cancer 2012 [34]. The trial recruited 1381 patients (1312 evaluable), and the results of a planned second interim analysis based on 551 deaths were presented. The two CT regimens were of similar efficacy. With a median follow-up exceeding 4 years the median PFS was 14 months in both trial arms, and the median OS was 32 months for TcP versus 38 months for TAP (HR 1.01). A higher percentage of patients on TcP were able to complete all seven planned courses of treatment (69% vs 62%). The toxicity rates favored TcP, which was less toxic except for neutropenia; 79% versus 52%. However, the incidence of neutropenic fever was similar for both regimens; 6% versus 7%. These results indicate that TcP was not inferior to and was less toxic than TAP.

An Italian and a Japanese trials compared adjuvant CAP CT with adjuvant pelvic EBRT [35, 36]. The Italian study randomized 345 (340 evaluable) patients with endometrioid or adenosquamous carcinoma and FIGO 1988 stage IC grade 3 or stage IIA to IIB grade 3 with ≥50% myometrial invasion or FIGO stage III (67% of patients had stage III EC) [35]. The Japanese trial randomized 475 women with stage IC to IIIC with 50% MI or greater; in this trial most patients had early disease stage and many had at most intermediate risk factors [36]. Both studies failed to show superiority of CT.

A pivotal study, GOG-122, changed opinions about CT of EC among many gynecologic oncologists [37]. Patients with FIGO 1988 stage III or IV EC of any histology were randomized to CT (AP every 3 weeks for seven cycles, followed by one cycle of cisplatin) or whole abdominal irradiation (WAI; 30 Gy in 20 fractions, with an additional 15 Gy pelvic boost) after surgical staging and optimal tumor resection (no single site of residual tumor greater than 2 cm). The trial recruited 422 (396 evaluable) patients, of whom 194 were allocated to CT and 202 to WAI. Both PFS and OS were significantly better for patients in the CT arm. The results were presented and analyzed for significance adjusted for stage, which is unusual for randomized studies, and has been criticized. The unadjusted Kaplan-Meier estimates for 5-year PFS were 42% versus 38%, and for OS 53% versus 42% in the CT and WAI arm, respectively. This should be compared with the adjusted values of 50% versus 38% and 55% versus 42%. The authors did not present P values for the unadjusted results. The treatment effect was consistent in subgroup analyses according to stage, substage, age, and residual disease status. An explanation for the difference in unadjusted OS despite the small difference in unadjusted PFS may be that second-line treatments could have a greater efficacy in those patients that had no previous irradiation. Grade 3 and 4 adverse effects (particularly hematologic, gastrointestinal, cardiac, and neurologic) were significantly more common in the CT arm. Treatment may have contributed to the death of five patients in the WAI arm and eight patients assigned to CT. The use of WAI in this setting has been debated as the dose and volume were not suitable in this patient population. Supposing that results were not caused by WAI worsening survival, CT still improved survival in this group of fairly advanced EC.

Based on the results of GOG-122 [37] the Leuven group recently suggested neoadjuvant CT with 3–4 courses of TcP and interval debulking surgery as a new treatment algorithm in stage IV endometrial cancer with transperitoneal spread [38]. The response rate to neoadjuvant CT according to RECIST among 30 patients was 74% with 7% complete responses. Patients with progressive disease (7%) were not operated. Twenty-eight patients underwent surgery, of which 86% had optimal tumor reduction to ≤1 cm tumor residuals; 92% of those had no remaining macroscopic tumor. Fourteen percent were considered inoperable. The median PFS and OS were 13 and 24 months, respectively.

Chemotherapy and Radiotherapy Combined

Two small randomized studies of EBRT versus combined EBRT and CT have been published (Table 2). In the historical GOG-34 published in 1990 [39] sequential adjuvant EBRT followed by single agent doxorubicin (A) was compared with EBRT alone in 224 patients (only 181 evaluable). Eligible patients had FIGO 1988 stage I and II (occult) EC, with one or more of the following high-risk features: ≥50% myometrial invasion, pelvic or para-aortic metastases, cervical extension (occult), or adnexal metastases. After EBRT patients were randomized to observation or to A 45 mg/m^2. The study was terminated prematurely because of slow recruitment and was flawed as 27% of women randomized to CT did not receive it, and many patients were lost to follow-up. No significant differences in OS or PFS were found. The authors concluded that the study was inconclusive due to small sample size and protocol violations. A randomized Finnish study compared split-course pelvic

EBRT (2x28 Gy separated by a pause of 3 weeks) with EBRT combined with one course of CT (cyclophosphamide 500 mg/m^2 + epirubicin (E) 60 mg/m^2 + P 50 mg/m^2) given before EBRT, one in the radiation pause, and one after EBRT [40]. Eligible patients had FIGO 1988 stage IA–B grade 3 or IC–IIIA grade 1–3. No significant survival difference could be found (age-adjusted HR 1.21; 95% CI 0.56–2.65), while more toxicity was reported in the combination arm, most notably severe bowel toxicity 9.5% versus 2.8%. This trial again is inconclusive because of the small sample size. It is also difficult to interpret because of a historical split-course EBRT schedule.

The Nordic Society of Gynecologic Oncology (NSGO) in collaboration with the European Organization for the Treatment and Research on Cancer (EORTC) compared sequential adjuvant EBRT and CT with EBRT in 383 patients (378 evaluable) [41]. Various CT combinations were used, mainly AP or EP (83%), but also TcP (10%), EcP (4%) and TEcP (3%) given after EBRT (69%) or before EBRT (17%; 4% unknown). This trial was the first to show a significant 7% increase in 5-year PFS with the addition of CT to EBRT from 72% to 79%; HR 0.64 (95% CI 0.41–0.99; P=0.04), but no significant difference in overall survival. The EORTC/NSGO trial was published together with the ILIADE-III study from the Italian MaNGO group. In the pooled data analysis with ILIADE-III (157 patients, for a combined total of 534 evaluable patients), results were similar, with a statistically significant difference in 5-year PFS favoring the combined arm: 78% for combined EBRT+CT versus 69% for EBRT alone, HR 0.63 (95% CI 0.44–0.89; P=0.009), but only a trend for improved 5-year OS (82% versus 75%, HR 0.63; 95% CI 0.46–1.03; P=0.07). For cancer-specific survival the difference was significant 87% versus 78%, HR 0.55 (95% CI 0.35–0.88; P=0.01). In the NSGO/EORTC trial, there was one treatment related death 3 months after randomization in the radiation arm. No further details were available. There were eight serious adverse events (SAE) in the CT+EBRT arm and one in the EBRT arm. All SAEs resolved after appropriate treatment. In the MaNGO trial no treatment related death was registered. It should be noted that although NSGO/EORTC and GOG-122 trials both showed a PFS benefit with CT for the overall trial populations, neither showed a trend for PFS or OS benefit from adjuvant CT for the subpopulations of patients with serous or clear cell tumors, although these were few in number (n=140 in NSGO/EORTC and n=100 in GOG-122). The hazard ratios for PFS and OS with CT were 0.91 and 1.02 for patients with serous or clear cell cancer in GOG-122, and 0.83 and 0.94, respectively, in the NSGO/EORTC trial. However, the GOG have analyzed their trials of

CT in patients with advanced or metastatic EC [42]. They found no evidence that serous or clear cell carcinomas responded differently to CT than endometrioid carcinomas. The problem is that these tumors comprise rather small subgroups in the trials leading to inconclusive results. Thus, there is a need to establish the efficacy of adjuvant CT for serous and clear cell cancers in separate randomized trials.

The Radiation Therapy Oncology Group (RTOG) have published a phase II study (RTOG-9708) of combined adjuvant pelvic EBRT (45 Gy + vaginal brachytherapy) with concomitant P (chemoradiotherapy) on days 1 and 28, followed by four courses of TP at 4-week intervals [43]. Patients with grade 2 or 3 endometrial adenocarcinoma with either >50% myometrial invasion, cervical stromal invasion, or pelvic-confined extra-uterine disease were eligible. This treatment was feasible with excellent loco-regional control suggesting additive effects of CT and radiation. Distant metastases, however, continued to occur in more advanced-stage patients.

Ongoing and Planned Trials

Ongoing trials investigating the roles of adjuvant CT, radiation therapy and combinations of CT and radiation therapy are the PORTEC-3 [44], GOG-249 [45] and GOG-258 [46] trials (see Table 6.5). The international randomized PORTEC-3 trial [44] is based on the RTOG phase II study [43]. Patients with high-risk EC (FIGO 2009 stage IA grade 3 LVSI+; stage IB grade 3; stage II; stage IIIA or IIIC ; stage IIIB (if parametrial invasion); or serous or clear cell histology of stage IA (with myometrial invasion), stage IB, stage II or III disease after surgery with no residual macroscopic tumor are randomized to pelvic adjuvant EBRT or chemoradiotherapy followed by CT. PORTEC has substituted TP used in the RTOG pilot [43] with TcP. The primary end points are OS and relapse-free survival (RFS) at 5 years. Secondary end points are quality of life, severe treatment related morbidity, rate of vaginal or pelvic relapse, and rate of distant metastases. The trial uses a uniform treatment schedule starting both treatments modalities early. It includes upfront pathology review to ensure that only patients with true high-risk tumors are included. Quality of life assessments are registered to establish short- and long-term toxicities and their impact on the patient´s daily life. Patient accrual is well underway and the study is expected to soon be completed.

Table 2. Randomized studies on adjuvant chemotherapy in early endometrial cancer

Reference	Study population	Control arm	Experimental arm	Outcome
Randall 2006 (37)	St II-IV of any histology, no postop tumor >2 cm without hematogenous or inguinal lymph node metastases	N=202; WAI 30 Gy + pelvic EBRT 15 Gy ± PA boost	N=194; doxorubicin 60 mg/m^2 + cisplatin 50 mg/m^2 every 3 weeks x 7 + cisplatin 50 mg/m^2 x 1	5-year OS adjusted for stage Control arm 42% Experimental arm 55% 5-year PFS adjusted for stage Control arm 38% Experimental arm 50%
Morrow 1990 (39)	FIGO st I-II (occult) all grades, and ≥1 of: ≥50% MI, PN+, PAN+, cervical invasion (occult), or adnexal mets	N=89 Pelvic EBRT 50 Gy ± PA EBRT	N=92 EBRT+doxorubicin 45 mg/m^2 to maximal cumulated dose of 400 (500) mg/m^2	5-year OS Approximately 60% in both study arms
Maggi 2006 (35)	FIGO st IC gr 3 or stage IIA-B gr 3 with ≥50% MI or FIGO st III non-serous/non-clear cell carcinoma	N=166 Pelvic EBRT 45-50 Gy ± PA EBRT 45 Gy	N=174 Cyclophosphamide 600 mg/m^2 + doxorubicin 45 mg/m^2 + cisplatin 50 mgm^2 every 4 weeks 4 weeks x 5	5-year OS Control arm 69% Experimental arm 66% 5-year PFS Control arm 63% Experimental arm 63%
Susumu 2008 (36)	FIGO st IC–IIIC endometrioid carcinoma and ≥50% MI and <75 years old	N=192 Pelvic EBRT 45-50 Gy ± PA EBRT ±VBT	N=193 Cyclophosphamide 333 mg/m^2 + doxorubicin 40 mg/m^2 + cisplatin 50 mg/m^2 every 4 weeks x ≥3	5-year OS Control arm 85% Experimental arm 87% 5-year PFS Control arm 84% Experimental arm 82%

Reference	Study population	Control arm	Experimental arm	Outcome
Hogberg 2010 (41)	Stage I, II, IIIA , IIIC and ≥ 1 of: grade 3, ≥50% MI, or DNA non-diploidy Stage I-III Serous/clear cell carcinoma	N=267 Pelvic EBRT ≥44 Gy ±VBT	n=267; Pelvic EBRT ≥44 Gy ± VBT, doxorubicin 50 mg/m^2 or epirubicin 75 mg/m^2 + cisplatin 50– 75 mg/m^2 (83%) or other regimens in 17% every 3–4 weeks × 3–4 (1/3 had chemotherapy before EBRT)	5-year OS Stage I–III serous/clear cell carcinoma Control arm 75% Experimental arm 82% 5-year PFS Control arm 69% Experimental arm 78%
Kuoppala 2008 (40)	Stage IA–B grade 3 or stage IC–IIIA grade 1–3	n=72; Pelvic EBRT 28 Gy in 2 courses with 3 weeks' pause between	n=84; cyclophosphamide 500 mg/m2 + epirubicin 60 mg/m2 + cisplatin 50 mg/m2 course 1 + pelvic EBRT 28 Gy + chemo course 2 + pelvic EBRT 28 Gy + chemo course 3	5-year CSS Control arm 85% Experimental arm 82%

CT: Chemotherapy, EBRT: external beam radiotherapy, FIGO: International Federation of Gynecology and Obstetrics, MI: Myometrial infiltration, Gy: Gray, PA: Para-aortic, PFS: Progression-free survival, PAN+: Para-aortal lymph node metastases, PN+: Pelvic lymph node metastases, WAI: Whole abdominal irradiation, OS: Overall survival.

GOG-249 is a randomized trial comparing EBRT alone with vaginal brachytherapy and 3 cycles of TcP; primary endpoint is RFS [45]. Eligible patients have stage I or II EC with high-intermediate or high-risk factors; recruitment is fast and the target of 562 patients may be reached in 2013. GOG-258, the companion trial for advanced stage EC is comparing 6 cycles of TcP alone with the same combined CT+EBRT schedule as in PORTEC-3. Eligible patients have optimally debulked stage III-IVA EC [46]. Finally, the ENGOT-EN2-DGCG-trial has recently started [47]. Patients with node-negative (LA required) stage I grade 3 or stage II endometrioid adencarcinoma or stage I-II clear cell, serous or squamous carcinoma stage I-II will be randomized to six courses of TcP versus observation. Vaginal brachytherapy is optional in both arms.

These trials will be able to answer many of the present questions and controversies regarding optimal use and optimal schedules of adjuvant therapy for women with high-risk and high-intermediate risk EC.

Targeted Drugs

The biologic characterization of individual tumors will in the near future be increasingly used to choose targeted compounds for treatment (personalized medicine) [48]. Targeted drugs have still only shown modest effects in EC. The studies have, however, been done treating patient groups that was not selected with respect to the molecular target aimed at by the substance at test [49] . There is a great risk to miss clinically important effects in such studies. If the target exists in 25% of the patients in a phase-II study and there is a 30% response rate only among those patients, the response rate for the whole study population would be only 7.5%. This may cause rejection of potentially active compounds. If trastuzumab combined with CT had been tested without pre-selection of patients with HER-2/neu–positive breast cancers [50], such a study would have required almost 24,000 randomly assigned patients to demonstrate a 1-year survival improvement of 2.4% [51]. Unfortunately, the emergence of predictive tests for targeted drugs often lags behind the introduction of new drugs.

The signal pathways that at present have been targeted in clinical trials in endometrial cancer is the inhibition of EGFR, VEGFR, and

PI3K/PTEN/AKT/mTOR signal pathways [52], but several other candidates exist [9, 52].

Conclusion

Lately CT has emerged as a primary treatment alternative in both advanced and early endometrial cancer. The most active drugs are anthracyclines, platinum drugs, and taxanes. Although rather high response rates are achieved, unfortunately PFS and OS are only moderately prolonged. New insights into the molecular mechanisms of tumor evolution will hopefully lead to better systemic treatments with targeted substances. The combination of CT and radiotherapy seems promising as adjuvant therapy in high-risk endometrial cancer and seems to be more effective than radiotherapy alone. However, we do not know if adequate CT only would be equally effective. GOG-258 addresses this question in advanced endometrial cancer with optimally debulked disease by comparing CT with paclitaxel and carboplatin versus external beam radiotherapy with concomitant cisplatin followed by paclitaxel and carboplatin.

References

[1] Ferlay, J; Shin, HR; Bray, F; Forman, D; Mathers, C; Parkin, DM. Estimates of worldwide burden of cancer in 2008: GLOBOCAN 2008. *International Journal of Cancer*, 2010, 127(12), 2893-917.

[2] Howlader, N; Noone, AM; Krapcho, M; Garshell, J; Neyman, N; Altekruse, SF;et al.. (eds). *SEER Cancer Statistics Review*, 1975-2010, National Cancer Institute. Bethesda, MD. Available from http://seer.cancer.gov/csr/1975_2010/, based on November 2012 SEER data submission, posted to the SEER web site, April 2013. 2013.

[3] Engholm, G; Ferlay, J; Christensen, N; Johannesen, TB; Klint, Å; Køtlum, JE; et al. *NORDCAN: Cancer Incidence, Mortality, Prevalence and Survival in the Nordic Countries*, Version 5.3 (25.04.2013). Association of the Nordic Cancer Registries. Danish Cancer Society. Available from http://www.ancr.nu.

[4] Creasman, WT; Odicino, F; Maisonneuve, P; Quinn, MA; Beller, U; Benedet, JL; et al. Carcinoma of the corpus uteri. FIGO 26th Annual Report on the Results of Treatment in Gynecological Cancer. *International Journal of Gynaecology and Obstetrics*, 2006, 95 Suppl 1, S105-43.

[5] Heintz, AP; Odicino, F; Maisonneuve, P; Quinn, MA; Benedet, JL; Creasman, WT; et al. Carcinoma of the ovary. FIGO 26th Annual Report on the Results of Treatment in Gynecological Cancer. *International Journal of Gynaecology and Obstetrics*, 2006, 95 Suppl 1, S161-92.

[6] Landrum, LM; Moore, KN; Myers, TK; Lanneau, GS Jr; McMeekin, DS; Walker, JL; et al. Stage IVB endometrial cancer: does applying an ovarian cancer treatment paradigm result in similar outcomes? A case-control analysis. *Gynecologic Oncology*, 2009, 112(2), 337-41.

[7] Bokhman, JV. Two pathogenetic types of endometrial carcinoma. *Gynecologic Oncology*, 1983, 15(1), 10-7.

[8] Bansal, N; Yendluri, V; Wenham, RM. The molecular biology of endometrial cancers and the implications for pathogenesis, classification, and targeted therapies. *Cancer Control: Journal of the Moffitt Cancer Center*, 2009, 16(1), 8-13.

[9] Engelsen, IB; Akslen, LA; Salvesen, HB. Biologic markers in endometrial cancer treatment. *APMIS: Acta Pathologica, Microbiologica, et Immunologica Scandinavica*, 2009, 117(10), 693-707.

[10] Kong, A; Johnson, N; Kitchener, HC; Lawrie, TA. Adjuvant radiotherapy for stage I endometrial cancer: an updated Cochrane systematic review and meta-analysis. *Journal of the National Cancer Institute*, 2012, 104(21), 1625-34.

[11] McMeekin, DS. Where is the future of endometrial cancer therapy? *Annals of Oncology*, 2009, 20(11), 1757-61.

[12] Creasman, WT; Morrow, CP; Bundy, BN; Homesley, HD; Graham, JE; Heller, PB. Surgical pathologic spread patterns of endometrial cancer. A Gynecologic Oncology Group Study. *Cancer*, 1987, 60(8 Suppl), 2035-41.

[13] Mariani, A; Dowdy, SC; Cliby, WA; Gostout, BS; Jones, MB; Wilson, TO; et al. Prospective assessment of lymphatic dissemination in endometrial cancer: a paradigm shift in surgical staging. *Gynecologic Oncology*, 2008, 109(1), 11-8.

[14] Pecorelli, S. Revised FIGO staging for carcinoma of the vulva, cervix, and endometrium. *International Journal of Gynecology and Obstetrics*, 2009, 105(2), 103-4.

[15] Humber, CE; Tierney, JF; Symonds, RP; Collingwood, M; Kirwan, J; Williams, C; et al. Chemotherapy for advanced, recurrent or metastatic endometrial cancer: a systematic review of Cochrane collaboration. *Annals of Oncology*, 2007, 18(3), 409-20.

[16] Temkin, SM; Fleming, G. Current treatment of metastatic endometrial cancer. *Cancer Control: Journal of the Moffitt Cancer Center*, 2009, 16(1), 38-45.

[17] Aapro, MS. Doxorubicin versus doxorubicin and cisplatin in endometrial carcinoma: definitive results of a randomised study (55872) by the EORTC Gynaecological Cancer Group. *Annals of Oncology*, 2003, 14(3), 441-8.

[18] Thigpen, JT; Brady, MF; Homesley, HD; Malfetano, J; DuBeshter, B; Burger, RA; et al. Phase III trial of doxorubicin with or without cisplatin in advanced endometrial carcinoma: a gynecologic oncology group study. *Journal of Clinical Oncology*, 2004, 22(19), 3902-8.

[19] Muggia, FM; Blessing, JA; Sorosky, J; Reid, GC. Phase II trial of the pegylated liposomal doxorubicin in previously treated metastatic endometrial cancer: a Gynecologic Oncology Group study. *Journal of Clinical Oncology*, 2002, 20(9), 2360-4.

[20] Homesley, HD; Blessing, JA; Sorosky, J; Reid, G; Look, KY. Phase II trial of liposomal doxorubicin at 40 mg/m^2 every 4 weeks in endometrial carcinoma: a Gynecologic Oncology Group Study. *Gynecologic Oncology*, 2005, 98(2), 294-8.

[21] Balbi, G; Visconti, S; Monteverde, A; Manganaro, MA; Cardone, A. Liposomal doxorubicin: a phase II trial. *Acta Bio-Medica*, 2007, 78(3), 210-3.

[22] Pujade-Lauraine, E; Wagner, U; Aavall-Lundqvist, E; Gebski, V; Heywood, M; Vasey, PA; et al. Pegylated liposomal Doxorubicin and Carboplatin compared with Paclitaxel and Carboplatin for patients with platinum-sensitive ovarian cancer in late relapse. *Journal of Clinical Oncology*, 2010, 28(20), 3323-9.

[23] du Bois, A; Pfisterer, J; Burchardi, N; Loibl, S; Huober, J; Wimberger, P; et al. Combination therapy with pegylated liposomal doxorubicin and carboplatin in gynecologic malignancies: a prospective phase II study of

the Arbeitsgemeinschaft Gynaekologische Onkologie Studiengruppe Ovarialkarzinom (AGO-OVAR) and Kommission Uterus (AGO-K-Ut). *Gynecologic Oncology*, 2007, 107(3), 518-25.

Pignata, S; Scambia, G; Pisano, C; Breda, E; Di Maio, M; Greggi, S; et al. A multicentre phase II study of carboplatin plus pegylated liposomal doxorubicin as first-line chemotherapy for patients with advanced or recurrent endometrial carcinoma: the END-1 study of the MITO (Multicentre Italian Trials in Ovarian Cancer and Gynecologic Malignancies) group. *British Journal of Cancer*, 2007, 96(11), 1639-43.

[24] Fleming, GF; Brunetto, VL; Cella, D; Look, KY; Reid, GC; Munkarah, AR; et al. Phase III trial of doxorubicin plus cisplatin with or without paclitaxel plus filgrastim in advanced endometrial carcinoma: a Gynecologic Oncology Group Study. *Journal of Clinical Oncology*, 2004, 22(11), 2159-66.

[25] Hoskins, PJ; Swenerton, KD; Pike, JA; Wong, F; Lim, P; Acquino-Parsons, C; et al. Paclitaxel and carboplatin, alone or with irradiation, in advanced or recurrent endometrial cancer: a phase II study. *Journal of Clinical Oncology*, 2001, 19(20), 4048-53.

[26] Sorbe, B; Andersson, H; Boman, K; Rosenberg, P; Kalling, M. Treatment of primary advanced and recurrent endometrial carcinoma with a combination of carboplatin and paclitaxel-long-term follow-up. *International Journal of Gynecological Cancer*, 2008, 18(4), 803-8.

[27] Akram, T; Maseelall, P; Fanning, J. Carboplatin and paclitaxel for the treatment of advanced or recurrent endometrial cancer. *American Journal of Obstetrics and Gynecology*, 2005, 192(5), 1365-7.

[28] Michener, CM; Peterson, G; Kulp, B; Webster, KD; Markman, M. Carboplatin plus paclitaxel in the treatment of advanced or recurrent endometrial carcinoma. *Journal of Cancer Research and Clinical Oncology*, 2005, 131(9), 581-4.

[29] Scudder, SA; Liu, PY; Wilczynski, SP; Smith, HO; Jiang, C; Hallum, AV 3rd; et al. Paclitaxel and carboplatin with amifostine in advanced, recurrent, or refractory endometrial adenocarcinoma: a phase II study of the Southwest Oncology Group. *Gynecologic Oncology*, 2005, 96(3), 610-5.

[30] Arimoto, T; Nakagawa, S; Yasugi, T; Yoshikawa, H; Kawana, K; Yano, T; et al. Treatment with paclitaxel plus carboplatin, alone or with

irradiation, of advanced or recurrent endometrial carcinoma. *Gynecologic Oncology*, 2007, 104(1), 32-5.

[31] Nomura, H; Aoki, D; Takahashi, F; Katsumata, N; Watanabe, Y; Konishi, I; et al. Randomized phase II study comparing docetaxel plus cisplatin, docetaxel plus carboplatin, and paclitaxel plus carboplatin in patients with advanced or recurrent endometrial carcinoma: a Japanese Gynecologic Oncology Group study (JGOG2041). *Annals of Oncology*, 2011, 22(3), 636-42.

[32] Aoki, D. Completion of patient enrollment to JGOG2043 a randomized phase III trial for endometrial cancer. *JGOG International*. 2012, Sep (no. 7), 2-3. Available from http://www.jgog.gr.jp/en/newsletter/pdf/ JGOG_ Inter_No.7.pdf.

[33] Miller, D; Felicias; V.; Fleming; G.; Mannel; R.; Cohn; D.; Matsumoto;et al. Late-Breaking Abstract 1: Randomized phase III noninferiority trial of first line chemotherapy for metastatic or recurrent endometrial carcinoma: A Gynecologic Oncology Group study. *Gynecologic Oncology*, 2012, 125, 771.

[34] Maggi, R; Lissoni, A; Spina, F; Melpignano, M; Zola, P; Favalli, G; et al. Adjuvant chemotherapy vs radiotherapy in high-risk endometrial carcinoma: results of a randomised trial. *British Journal of Cancer*, 2006, 95(3), 266-71.

[35] Susumu, N; Sagae, S; Udagawa, Y; Niwa, K; Kuramoto, H; Satoh, S; et al. Randomized phase III trial of pelvic radiotherapy versus cisplatin-based combined chemotherapy in patients with intermediate- and high-risk endometrial cancer: a Japanese Gynecologic Oncology Group study. *Gynecologic Oncology*, 2008, 108(1), 226-33.

[36] Randall, ME; Filiaci, VL; Muss, H; Spirtos, NM; Mannel, RS; Fowler, J; et al. Randomized phase III trial of whole-abdominal irradiation versus doxorubicin and cisplatin chemotherapy in advanced endometrial carcinoma: a Gynecologic Oncology Group Study. *Journal of Clinical Oncology*, 2006, 24(1), 36-44.

[37] Vandenput, I; Van, Calster, B; Capoen, A; Leunen, K; Berteloot, P; Neven, P; et al. Neoadjuvant chemotherapy followed by interval debulking surgery in patients with serous endometrial cancer with transperitoneal spread (stage IV): a new preferred treatment? *British Journal of Cancer*, 2009, 101(2), 244-9.

[38] Morrow, CP; Bundy, BN; Homesley, HD; Creasman, WT; Hornback, NB; Kurman, R; et al. Doxorubicin as an adjuvant following surgery and radiation therapy in patients with high-risk endometrial carcinoma, stage I and occult stage II: a Gynecologic Oncology Group Study. *Gynecologic Oncology*, 1990, 36(2), 166-71.

[39] Kuoppala, T; Maenpaa, J; Tomas, E; Puistola, U; Salmi, T; Grenman, S; et al. Surgically staged high-risk endometrial cancer: randomized study of adjuvant radiotherapy alone vs. sequential chemo-radiotherapy. *Gynecologic Oncology*, 2008, 110(2), 190-5.

[40] Hogberg, T; Signorelli, M; de, Oliveira, CF; Fossati, R; Lissoni, AA; Sorbe, B; et al. Sequential adjuvant chemotherapy and radiotherapy in endometrial cancer--results from two randomised studies. *European Journal of Cancer*, 2010, 46(13), 2422-31.

[41] McMeekin, DS; Filiaci, VL; Thigpen, JT; Gallion, HH; Fleming, GF; Rodgers, WH; et al. The relationship between histology and outcome in advanced and recurrent endometrial cancer patients participating in first-line chemotherapy trials: a Gynecologic Oncology Group study. *Gynecologic Oncology*, 2007, 106(1), 16-22.

[42] Greven, K; Winter, K; Underhill, K; Fontenesci, J; Cooper, J; Burke, T. Final analysis of RTOG 9708: adjuvant postoperative irradiation combined with cisplatin/paclitaxel chemotherapy following surgery for patients with high-risk endometrial cancer. *Gynecologic Oncology*, 2006, 103(1), 155-9.

[43] PORTEC-3 trial. Available from http://clinicaltrials.gov/ct2/show/NCT00411138.

[44] GOG-249 trial. Available from http://clinicaltrials.gov/ct2/show/NCT00807768.

[45] GOG-258 trial. Available from http://clinicaltrials.gov/ct2/show/NCT00942357.

[46] ENGOT-EN2-DGCG trial. Available from http://clinicaltrials.gov/ct2/show/NCT01244789.

[47] Sood, AK; Coleman, RL. Targeted therapy in gynecologic oncology: biology, strategy, and assessment. *Gynecologic Oncology*, 2010, 116(2), 155-6.

[48] Bergh, J. Quo vadis with targeted drugs in the 21st century? *Journal of Clinical Oncology*, 2009, 27(1), 2-5.

[49] Slamon, DJ; Leyland-Jones, B; Shak, S; Fuchs, H; Paton, V; Bajamonde, A; et al. Use of chemotherapy plus a monoclonal antibody against HER2 for metastatic breast cancer that overexpresses HER2. *The New England Journal of Medicine*, 2001, 344(11), 783-92.

[50] Simon, R; Maitournam, A. Evaluating the efficiency of targeted designs for randomized clinical trials. *Clinical Cancer Research*, 2004, 10(20), 6759-63.

[51] Dedes, KJ; Wetterskog, D; Ashworth, A; Kaye, SB; Reis-Filho, JS. Emerging therapeutic targets in endometrial cancer. *Nature Reviews Clinical Oncology*, 2011, 8(5), 261-71.

In: Endometrial Cancer
Editors: I. Diaz-Padilla, J. Garcia-Donas
ISBN: 978-1-63321-323-4

Chapter VIII

Systemic Chemotherapy: Endometrial Cancer

John A. Green*
Institute of Translational Medicine,
University of Liverpool,
Liverpool, UK

Abstract

Cytotoxic chemotherapy with cisplatin or carboplatin, doxorubicin and paclitaxel in doublet form provides control of advanced and recurrent disease for about 12 months. There is also more limited evidence for the use of adjuvant chemotherapy in high risk subgroups with no universal agreement on patient selection. Molecular subtyping of endometrial cancer is still under development, but there is evidence the proportion of serous tumours may have been underestimated in the past. Hormone therapy may be of use in receptor positive patients, and carboplatin and paclitaxel chemotherapy in patients relapsing after local treatment is emerging as the standard of care. However, targeted therapy has produced modest responses to date with no evidence of a contribution to prolongation of survival, but offers promise of disease control with less systemic toxicity.

* E-mail: j.a.green@liverpool.ac.uk; Tel.: 0044 151 482 7793; Fax: 0044 151 482 7621.

Introduction

There has been considerable progress in the chemotherapy of endometrial cancer over the last 10 years, although compared to other gynaecological cancers such as those arising, or thought to arise in the ovary, chemotherapy for advanced or recurrent endometrial cancer has been slow to develop for a number of reasons. Many patients have slowly growing disease without a rapid onset of symptoms, the patient population is older, and many of the type 1 cancers have co-morbidities such as obesity, diabetes and cardiac problems which impair the ability to administer full doses of conventional chemotherapy.

For some of the low grade cancers, which largely correspond to the endometrioid subtypes, hormone treatments with hyroxyprogesterone acetate, megestrol and tamoxifen have been employed. More recently as part of the PARAGON phase II trial, anastrazole has been used [1, 2]. Following on from the universal use of ER and PR assessment in breast cancer, semiquantitative measurement has been applied to endometrial cancer diagnostic biopsies to aid patient selection for these treatments, although there is no standardization of methodology across European centres. A further problem is that the available tissue may antedate the clinical picture of advanced disease by several years in the case of recurrent disease, and a view has to be taken on the feasibility and risk associated with re-biopsy in an attempt to individualise drug selection, instead of relying on an empirical selection of treatment based on historical characterization of the tumour.

From single agent studies in the 1990's, cisplatin and doxorubicin emerged as the most effective agents, although renal and cardiac toxicity limited their application to all endometrial cancer patients. Attempts to add a third drug such as paclitaxel led to marginal improvement in efficacy, but increasing toxicity did not lead to triplet therapy becoming widely accepted outside the US [3]. As in many other solid tumours, carboplatin has gradually come to replace cisplatin in combinations without significant loss of efficacy. Of the targeted therapies, uncertainty remains over the possible benefit of bevacizumab - in ovarian cancer the addition of this drug as concomitant with chemotherapy and maintenance has shown a survival gain in high risk subgroups such as those with incompletely debulked tumours [4]. Also, in cervical cancer GOG 240 has shown an overall survival benefit of 3.7 months [5], predominantly in those with small volume residual disease and pelvic disease, but at a high cost in terms of fistula formation, as might be expected in patients with prior radiation therapy. In endometrial cancer there have been no randomized studies published to take forward the study of bevacizumab in relapsed disease. Many endometrial cancer patients have also received prior whole pelvic or vaginal vault brachytherapy, and in more recent years chemoradiation as described in Chapter 7 above, so concerns about fistula risk remain.

Review of the Randomised Studies of Chemotherapy for Advanced Disease

A systematic meta-analysis of 14 trials accruing between 1974 and 2005 was reported by Vale et al. in 2013 [6]. Single agent response rates of 7-19% were reported. The authors reviewed eight of the trials which entered 1571 patients and randomized between more intensive and less intensive chemotherapy. This analysis showed that the overall survival (OS) (HR 0.86 95%CI 0.77-0.96) and PFS (HR 0.82 CI 0.74-0.90) were both longer when the more intensive regimens were used. There were extensive differences in prior therapy and treatment regimens in these studies which limited the interpretation of the analysis. However, serious acute toxicities were also more common in women randomized to the more intensive regimens. The phase III trial data is summarised in Table I.

JGOG 2041 [7] was a randomised phase II study reported in 2011 which compared the doublets docetaxel plus cisplatin, docetaxel plus carboplatin and paclitaxel plus carboplatin.

There was no evidence that any particular chemotherapy doublet was better or worse than another, and this trial has contributed to carboplatin and paclitaxel becoming the standard of care in Europe. The preliminary results of GOG 209 [8] have shown that this regimen is as effective and less toxic than the cisplatin, doxorubicin and paclitaxel triplet.

There have been no comparative trials with endocrine therapy [1], which may be used in ER or PR positive patients where a rapid response is not required, and is also often an appropriate choice in elderly patients on account of favourable toxicity compared to chemotherapy. Clinicians have interpreted the overall phase II and III trial data by largely employing carboplatin and paclitaxel in patients to treat advanced disease in the absence of significant diabetes or cardiac disease. Doxorubicin and cisplatin are more frequently used as second line therapy, although the trial data also supports their use as first line therapy.

Table 1. Randomised trials in advanced endometrial cancer comparing one drug with > one drug, a doublet with > two drugs or a triplet with four drugs. Key: mel melphalan, meg megestrol, cyclo cyclophosphamide, cis cisplatin, dox doxorubicin, mtx methotrexate, vin vinblastine

Study		Randomised pts	Median age (range)	Overall response %	Median PFS (m)	Median OS (m)
Horton 1982	Meg, cyclo,dox +/- 5-FU	131	64 (37-85)	23 vs 13	NR	NR
Aapro 2003	Dox +/- cis	177	63 (40-76)	17 vs 43	7 vs 8	7 vs 9
Cohen 1984	Mel, 5-FU, meg vs dox, cyclo, 5-FU, meg	295	63 (33-82)	38 vs 36	6 vs 5	11 vs 10
Edmons on 1987	Cis vs cis,dox, cyclo	30	65 (41-79)	21 vs 31	1.8 vs 2.9	7.4 vs 6.6
Fleming 2004	Dox, cis vs dox, cis, paclitaxel + filgrastim	273	(50-81)	34 vs 57	5.3 vs 8.3	12.3 vs 15.3
Long 2006	Dox, cyclo vs dox, cyclo, mtx, vin	28	66 (37-79)	26 vs 69	6.2 vs 6.9	6.2 vs 6.9
Thigpen 1994	Dox vs dox, cis	356	65 (36-90)	22 vs 30	22 vs 30	6.9 vs 7.3
Thigpen 2004	Dox vs dox,cis	281	65.5 (NS)	25 vs 42	25 vs 42	9.0 vs 9.2

Histology Specific Treatment

The ESMO clinical practice guidelines [9] make no recommendation on treatment of individual sub-types, but note that many existing studies such as PORTEC III, EORTC 55984 and 55991 contain patients with a range of histological subtypes, and some limited analyses may result from the outcome of these studies. In practice, many clinicians treat endometrial serous tumours in the same way as ovarian cancer in view of their morphological and molecular similarity, although the overall response rate and duration of remission in relapsed disease may be less than in the corresponding ovarian tumours. Similarly there is considerable variation in the chemotherapy treatment of carcinosarcoma, which most pathologists regard as an undifferentiated form of epithelial tumour, despite the terminology. One approach is to select the drugs according to the predominant histological component, based on a similar approach often employed in mixed tumours, which might lead to the use of doxorubicin in less differentiated tumours, and carboplatin based treatment in epithelial tumours. However, the increasing use of carboplatin and paclitaxel as the first line combination in endometrial cancer has reduced some of this practice variation.

Therefore, currently we do not have specific treatments for each histological subtype of endometrial cancer, but these categories are expected to themselves evolve over the next few years with the incorporation of molecular parameters.

Targeted Therapy

Following the demonstration that PTEN mutations were common in endometrial cancer leading to consequent activation of the PI3Kinase pathway, mTOR inhibitors were widely assessed in the early parts of this century. The results of these non- randomised single agent studies were fairly modest (reviewed in Dedes et al. [10]), with no complete responses and partial response rates less than 15%. Subsequent analyses of these pathways has shown this approach to be overly simplistic. In an approach designed to improve on this, one phase II study showed promising activity of dual TORC inhibition, which prevents feedback activation of the AKT pathway by the mTOR complex [11]. Other approaches to targeting of multiple components of this growth factor pathway are currently being explored including AKT, PI3K and MEK inhibitors [10]. As PTEN loss is associated with dysfunctional homologous repair, PARP inhibitors are also under investigation. EGFR and VEGFR inhibitors have also shown modest activity to date [12, 13] and other growth factor pathways including FGF seem appropriate ones to target.

One study of therapy combining mTOR and VEGF inhibition gave a median progression–free interval of 6 months and toxicity was considerable with 38% discontinuing therapy for this reason [14]. These results are modest with evidence of tumour response but times to progression in terms of months, which may reflect the absence of patient selection based on predictive markers. However, companion biomarkers have been difficult to define for the PI3kinase pathway, and most studies to date have been in unselected patients.

A further boost to the targeted therapy approach has been given by the TCGA analysis [15] of endometrial cancer published in mid-2013, which analysed the genomic, transcriptomic and proteomic characteristics of 373 tumours using array and sequencing based technologies. This recently published data has shown extensive abnormalities in a number of pathways, particularly the PI3K/AKT pathways, opening up several directed approaches. This paper also demonstrated was that there was molecular heterogeneity within the histological category of endometrioid tumours, and with the new WHO categorisation of endometrial cancer expected in April 2014, re-evaluation of existing series of tumours will be carried out. A key finding was that about 25% of the endometrioid tumours had profiles more like those of serous tumours [15]. It has been clear for some time that the molecular characteristics of Type 2 cancers such as p53 mutation and extensive copy number abnormalities are also present in a smaller proportion of type 1 cancers. However, the analysis of outcome groups based on cluster analysis shown in the main paper remains to be validated. Molecular heterogeneity both within tumours and within subtypes remains a problem.

Future Directions

It seems unlikely that further improvement can be achieved by conventional chemotherapeutic combinations alone. One interesting approach is AEZS-108 [16], a fusion molecule of LHRH and doxorubicin designed to target the LHRH receptors present in endometrial cancer. Combination of chemotherapy and PI3K pathway targeted tyrosine kinase inhibitors is also under investigation. Multi-pathway targeting is also possible with the range of molecules available, but early studies have led to concerns over toxicity.

Conclusion

Effective chemotherapy regimens are now available in endometrial cancer which have been validated in both the advanced and adjuvant settings. Hormone treatment has no value in the adjuvant setting, but can be incorporated into the treatment plan of advanced disease if appropriate receptors are identified and has the advantage of comparatively modest toxicity. Individualising the approaches described to the histological subtypes and molecular characteristics of the tumours is in progress.

References

[1] DeCruze SB and Green JA (2007) Hormone therapy for advanced and recurrent endometrial cancer – a systematic review. *Int. J. Gynecol. Oncol.*, 17(5): 964-78.

[2] PARAGON trial. http://www.anzgog.org.au/uploads/ ANZGOGTrial-Paragon.pdf (accessed 13.12.13)

[3] Fleming G. F., Brunetto V. L., Cella D. et al. (2004) Phase III trial of doxorubicin plus cisplatin with or without paclitaxel plus filgrastim in advanced endometrial carcinoma: a Gynecologic Oncology Group Study. *Journal of Clinical Oncology*, 22(11):2159-66.

[4] Perren T. J., Swart A. M., Pfisterer J. et al. (2011) A phase III trial of bevacizumab in ovarian cancer. *N. Engl. J. Med.*, 2011; 365:2484-2496.

[5] Monk B. J., Sill M. W., Gray H. J. et al. (2009) Phase II trial of bevacizumab in the treatment of persistent or recurrent squamous cell carcinoma of the cervix: a Gynecologic Oncology Group study. *J. Clin. Oncol.,* 27 1069-1074.

[6] Vale C. L., Tierney J., Bull S. J. and Symonds P. R. (2013) Chemotherapy for advanced , recurrent or metastatic endometrial carcinoma. Cochrane database of systematic reviews (4).

[7] Nomura H., Aoki D., Takahashi F. et al. (2011)Randomised phase II study comparing docetaxel plus cisplatin, docetaxel plus carboplatin, and paclitaxel plus carboplatin in patients with advanced or recurrent endometrial carcinoma: a Japanese Gynecologic Oncology Group Study (JGOG2041) *Annal. Oncol.*, 22(3): 636-42.

[8] Miller D., Filiaci V., Fleming G. et al. (2012) Randomized phase III non-inferiority trial of first line chemotherapy for metastatic or recurrent endometrial carcinoma: a Gynecologic Oncology Group study. *Gynecol. Oncol.*, 125:771-3.

[9] Colombo N., Preti E., Landoni F. et al. (2011) Endometrial cancer: ESMO clinical practice guidelines for diagnosis, treatment and follow-up. *Annal. Oncol.,* 22 (suppl. 6) vi35-39.

[10] Dedes K. J., Wetterskog D., Ashworth A. et al. (2011), Emerging therapeutic targets in endometrial cancer. *Nat. Rev. Clin. Oncol.*, 261-271.

[11] Shoji K., Odo K., Kashiyama T. et al. (2012) Genotype-dependent efficacy of a dual PI3K/mTOR inhibitor, NUP-BEZ and an mTOR inhibitor RAD 001 in endometrial carcinomas. *PloS ONE*, 7(5) 37431.
[12] Aghajianan C., Sill M. W., Darcy K. M. et al. (2011) Phase II trial of bevacizumab in recurrent or persistent endometrial cancer: a Gynecologic Oncology Group study. *J. Clin. Oncol.,* 29 (16) 2259-65.
[13] Leslie K. K., Sill M. W., Lankes H. A. et al. (2012) Lapatanib and prognostic value of EGFR mutations in Gynecologic Oncology Group phase II trial of persistent or recurrent endometrial cancer. *Gynecol. Oncol.,* 2012 127 (2) 345-350.
[14] Alvarez E. A., Brady W. E., Walker J. L. et al. (2013) Phase II study of combination bevacizumab and temsirolimus in the treatment of recurrent or persistent endometrial carcinoma: a Gynecologic Oncology Group Study. *Gynecologic Oncology*, 129 22-27.
[15] The Cancer Genome Atlas (TCGA) Research Network Integrated genomic characterization of endometrial carcinoma (2013) *Nature,* 497 67-73.
[16] Engel J., Emons G., Pinski J. and Schally A. V. (2012) AEZS-108; a targeted cytotoxic analog of LHRH for the treatment of cancers positive for LHRH receptors. *Expert Opin. Investig. Drugs,* (6) 891-9.

In: Endometrial Cancer
Editors: I. Diaz-Padilla, J. Garcia-Donas ISBN: 978-1-63321-323-4

Chapter IX

Molecular Targeted Therapies in Endometrial Cancer: Current Concepts and Future Challenges

***Shannon N. Westin*[1*] *and Russell R. Broaddus*[2]**
[1]Department of Gynecologic Oncology, University of Texas M. D. Anderson Cancer Center, Houston TX, US
[2]Department of Pathology, University of Texas M. D. Anderson Cancer Center, Houston TX, US

Abstract

The treatment of advanced and recurrent endometrial cancer is hampered by a paucity of effective agents and minimal durable response. Numerous potentially druggable molecular aberrations and the need for novel therapies have led to significant interest in the use of targeted agents in this disease. Although early results have been promising, targeted therapy has yet to reach its considerable potential in endometrial cancer. Challenges include paucity of tissue for testing, especially in

* Corresponding Author: Shannon N. Westin, M.D., M.P.H. Assistant Professor; Department of Gynecologic Oncology and Reproductive Medicine, Unit 1362, University of Texas M.D. Anderson Cancer Center, 1155 Herman Pressler, Houston, Texas 77030, (713) 794-4314, swestin@mdanderson.org.
Funding: NIH 2P50 CA098258-06 SPORE in Uterine Cancer. K12 CA088084 K12 Calabresi Scholar Award (SW).

metastasis, lack of predictive biomarkers, and appropriate trial design. Our growing understanding of the molecular context of endometrial tumors will continue to inform the development of rational clinical trials to incorporate targeted therapy into the standard treatment of endometrial cancer.

Introduction

The majority of early stage endometrial cancers confined to the uterus may be cured with current therapeutic approaches; however, patients with advanced stage or recurrent disease have dismal outcomes [1]. Further, there is a clear lack of Federal Drug Administration (FDA) approved treatments for this disease. These facts, combined with the growing documentation that a high proportion of endometrial cancers have molecular aberrations that can be targeted, provide the foundation for the rational evaluation of targeted agents for the treatment of endometrial cancer.

Molecular Aberrations in Endometrial Cancer

As understanding of tumorigenesis and molecular biology has grown, myriad pathways have been explored for their impact on the survival capabilities of cancer cells [2]. Interestingly, many of the pathways known to confer growth advantages to cancer cells are aberrant in endometrial cancer (Figure 1). Aberrations in these pathways appear to be dependent on the histologic type of endometrial cancer, indicating different mechanisms for cell growth and survival [3].

The endometrioid subtype of endometrial carcinoma is associated with numerous mutations affecting a variety of different pathways (Table 1). These tumors demonstrate potentially clinically significant alterations in the Phosphatidylinositol-3-Kinase(PI3K)/AKT pathway and the RAS/RAF pathway, in addition to amplifications in receptor tyrosine kinases (RTKs) that activate and interact with these pathways. PTEN aberrations, including loss of protein expression or mutation, are the most common in this subtype of endometrial carcinoma [4-7]. Mutations in *PI3KCA, PI3KR1*, and *FGFR2* are also common [8-12]. Uterine serous carcinomas have quite a different molecular profile from the endometrioid tumors (Table 2). This subtype is typically characterized by mutations in *TP53*, β-catenin, over-expression of HER2/neu, and wide-spread chromosomal copy number alterations [13-17]. Molecular alterations in the more rare non-endometrioid cell types, such as clear cell carcinoma and carcinosarcoma, are less well known. In general, they mirror what is found in the uterine serous population [16] (Table 2).

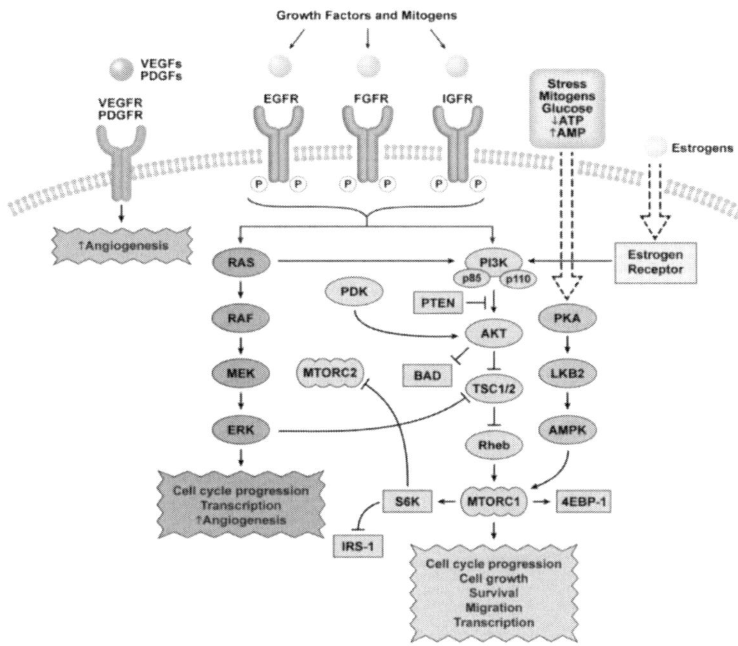

Figure 1. Relevant molecular pathways in endometrial cancer. Abbreviations: VEGF, Vascular Endothelial Growth Factor; VEGFR, Vascular Endothelial Growth Factor Receptor; PDGF, Platelet-derived Growth Factor; PDGFR, Platelet-derived Growth Factor Receptor; EGFR, Epidermal Growth Factor Receptor; FGFR2, Fibroblast Growth Factor Receptor 2; IGFR1, Insulin-like Growth Factor Receptor 1; ATP, Adenosine Triphosphate; ADP, Adenosine Diphosphate; RAS, V-Ki-ras2 Kirsten rat sarcoma viral oncogene homolog; RAF, mouse viral rapidly accelerated fibrosarcoma oncogene; MEK, Mitogen-activated protein kinase kinase; ERK, Mitogen-activated protein kinase; PDK, phosphoinositide-dependent kinase; BAD, Bcl-2-associated death promoter, TSC1/2, Tuberous sclerosis protein 1/2; PTEN, Phosphatase and Tensin Homolog Deleted on Chromosome 10; PI3K, Phosphatidylinositol 3 Kinase; AKT, v-akt murine thymoma viral oncogene homolog 1; mTORC1, mammalian Target of Rapamicin Complex 1; mTORC2, mammalian Target of Rapamicin Complex 2; S6K, Ribosomal protein S6 kinase; 4EBP-1, Eukaryotic translation initiation factor 4E binding protein 1; IRS-1, Insulin Receptor Substrate 1; PKA, Protein kinase A; LKB2, Liver kinase B1; AMPK, AMP-activated protein kinase.

Table 1. Frequency of common molecular aberrations in endometrioid type endometrial carcinoma

Alteration	Endometrioid (%)
PTEN protein loss (4,5,110)	80
PTEN mutation (7, 110)	30-50
PIK3CA mutation (8-10)	30-40
PIK3R1 mutation (11, 111)	43
AKT mutation (112, 113)	2-3
KRAS mutation (14, 64)	10-30
HRAS mutation (63)	7
IGFIR over-expression (83, 84)	78
FGFR2 mutation (12, 114)	12-16
EGFR over-expression (16, 115)	46
EGFR mutation	Unknown
HER2 over-expression (16, 115)	3-10
HER2 amplification (17, 116)	1
Beta catenin mutation (15, 117)	15-50
TP53 mutation (14, 118, 119)	0-20
E cadherin loss (15, 120, 121)	5-50
Microsatellite instability (14, 122, 123)	15-20

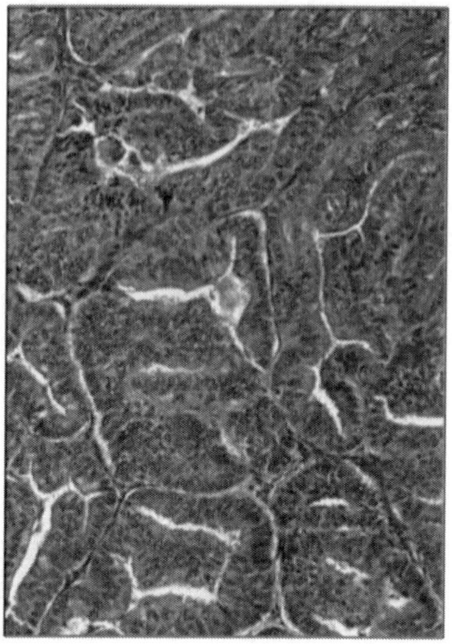

Abbreviations PTEN, Phosphatase and Tensin Homolog Deleted on Chromosome 10 ; PIK3CA, Phosphatidylinositol 3 Kinase, Catalytic, α Polypeptide ; PIK3RI, Phosphatidylinositol 3 Kinase, Regulatory Polypeptide ; AKT, v-akt murine thymoma viral oncogene homolog 1 ; KRAS, V-Ki-ras2 Kirsten rat sarcoma viral oncogene homolog ; IGFR1, Insulin-like Growth Factor Receptor 1 ; FGFR2, Fibroblast Growth Factor Receptor 2 ; EGFR, Epidermal Growth Factor Receptor ; HER, Human Epidermal Growth Factor Receptor.

PI3K/AKT Pathway

The PI3K/AKT pathway is a key regulator of cellular processes important to tumorigenesis including avoidance of apoptosis, proliferation, survival, and chemoresistance [18, 19]. The pathway is stimulated by nutrients and mitogens including insulin-like growth factor (IGF), epidermal growth factor (EGF), and fibroblast growth factor (FGF). These growth factors act through their respective receptor tyrosine kinases (RTKs) or G protein-coupled receptors to activate the PI3K heterodimer which is composed of two subunits, the p110 catalytic and the p85 regulatory subunit [19, 20]. In addition, cross-talk with the RAS/RAF, AMPK, and estrogen receptor pathways can also lead to the activation of PI3K and its downstream targets [21, 22].

Table 2. Frequency of common molecular aberrations in endometrial cancer of non-endometrioid histology

Alteration	Non-endometrioid(%)
PTEN protein loss (5, 110)	5
PTEN mutation (7, 110)	0-11
PIK3CA mutation (8, 124)	20
PIK3R1 mutation (11, 111)	12
AKT mutation (113)	0
KRAS mutation (14, 64)	0-10
HRAS mutation	unknown
IGFIR over-expression	unknown
FGFR2 mutation (12, 114)	1
EGFR over-expression (16, 115)	34
EGFR mutation (124)	0
HER2 over-expression (16, 115)	32
HER2 amplification (17, 116)	17
Beta catenin mutation (15)	0
TP53 mutation (14, 118, 125)	90
E cadherin loss (15, 121)	60-90
Microsatellite instability (14, 122, 123)	0-5

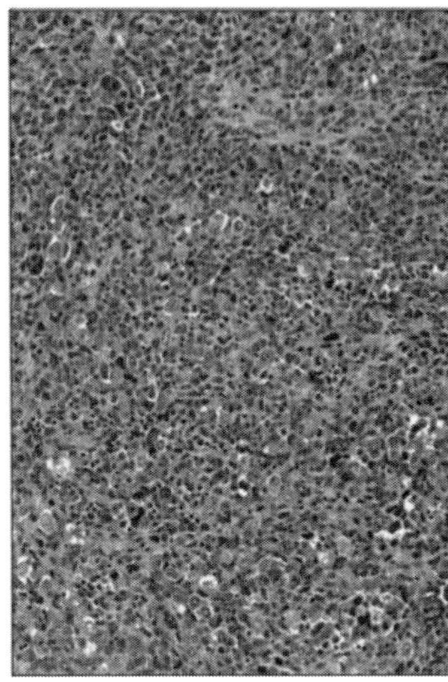

Abbreviations: PTEN, Phosphatase and Tensin Homolog Deleted on Chromosome 10 ; PIK3CA, Phosphatidylinositol 3 Kinase, Catalytic, α Polypeptide ; PIK3RI, Phosphatidylinositol 3 Kinase, Regulatory Polypeptide ; AKT, v-akt murine thymoma viral oncogene homolog 1 ; KRAS, V-Ki-ras2 Kirsten rat sarcoma viral oncogene homolog; IGFR1, Insulin-like Growth Factor Receptor 1 ; FGFR2, Fibroblast Growth Factor Receptor 2 ; EGFR, Epidermal Growth Factor Receptor ; HER, Human Epidermal Growth Factor Receptor.

PI3K acts to phosphorylate phosphatidylinositol 4,5- biphosphate (PIP2) to yield phosphatidylinositol 3,4,5- triphosphate (PIP3) [23]. Pleckstrin homology domain-containing proteins, including PDK1 and AKT, are recruited to the plasma membrane by PIP3 [24]. The tumor suppressors PTEN and INPP4B act to negatively regulate this process, converting PIP3 to PIP2. Once AKT is recruited to the plasma membrane, it undergoes phosphorylation by mammalian target of rapamycin (mTOR) complex 2 (mTORC2). Upon activation, AKT stimulates numerous downstream events, leading to proliferation, survival, and angiogenesis [18, 19]. A key action of AKT is to phosphorylate and inhibit the TSC complex, thus releasing the inhibition of mTORC1. mTORC1 is known to regulate metabolism and protein synthesis, leading to further tumorigenesis [25].

Targeting the PI3K/AKT Pathway in Endometrial Cancer

The numerous aberrations in the PI3K/AKT pathway found in endometrial cancer have generated a great deal of excitement for the therapeutic potential of agents targeting this pathway. Current options to target the PI3K/AKT pathway include inhibitors of mTOR, PI3K, and AKT or dual inhibitors of PI3K and mTOR. To date, the majority of trials featuring agents targeting this pathway have demonstrated only modest results. However, results have primarily been reported for trials of mTORC1 inhibitors (rapalogs). It may be that agents that target nodes higher in the pathway or multiple nodes are more effective at taking advantage of the molecular aberrations found in endometrial cancer.

mTOR Inhibition

In the preclinical setting, inhibition of mTOR leads to growth inhibition in endometrial cancer cell lines and xenograft models, particularly in those harboring aberrations in the PI3K/AKT pathway [26, 27]. Clinically, the success of mTOR inhibition as a single agent has been encouraging, but limited. The bulk of the trials completed in endometrial cancer have featured mTORC1 inhibitors, or rapalogues, including temsirolimus, everolimus, and ridaforolimus. These agents have achieved objective response rates ranging from 4 – 12%, with the highest success achieved in chemonaive endometrial cancer. Prolonged stable disease (SD) is more common, yielding clinical benefit rates from 29 - 57% [28-33]. Although promising, there is clearly progress necessary to yield a higher impact on survival in this disease. The failure of mTOR inhibition to live up to potential may be related to known feedback loops that exist within endometrial cancer. For example, mTORC2 is known to be negatively regulated by mTORC1 via S6K. The inhibition of mTORC1 allows for unhindered activation of AKT and subsequent resistance [34]. Crosstalk between the PI3K/AKT and RAS/RAF pathways may also contribute to resistance in the setting of single node inhibition. Increasing understanding of potential mechanisms for resistance has led to interest in targeting nodes higher in the PI3K/AKT pathway, as well as the combinatorial approaches across pathways including RAS/RAF and relevant receptor tyrosine kinases.

AKT Inhibition

Mutations in *AKT* are quite rare in endometrial cancer, but the increased signaling through this node has led to great excitement for incorporation of AKT inhibition into the treatment of this disease. In addition to known activity within the pathway, it appears that the activation of AKT is a major mechanism of resistance to anti-cancer therapies such as hormones and cytotoxic chemotherapy [35]. Further, the inhibition of AKT has led to reversal of chemotherapy resistance in endometrial cancer cell lines [36, 37]. This enthusiasm is somewhat tempered by the finding of increased signaling through receptor tyrosine kinases, including IGFIR and HER3, after inhibition of AKT [38]. AKT inhibition is achieved clinically through agents that compete for the ATP-binding site or bind AKT allosterically, preventing recruitment to the cell membrane. Agents such as perifostine and MK-2206 have shown promising ability to inhibit proliferation in cell lines [39, 40], but have shown modest activity in the clinical setting. A phase II trial of MK-2206 which stratified for PIK3CA mutations, achieved a 5% partial response (PR) rate and 33% of patients had SD at 8 weeks [41]. Early phase trials are ongoing with multiple competitive AKT inhibitors including AZD5363, GDC-0068, and GSK2141795.

PI3K Inhibition

Opportunities for the inhibition of PI3K include agents that inhibit all PI3K isoforms (pan-PI3K inhibitors) or inhibit only one isoform (isoform-selective PI3K inhibitors). The pan-PI3K inhibitors have demonstrated cancer cell line growth inhibition, including endometrial cancer [42-44]. In general, these agents are in early phase I trials in advanced solid tumors, although XL147 and BKM120 are under evaluation for endometrial cancer in the phase II setting. It is notable that pan-PI3K inhibitors are associated with significant toxicity including rash, nausea, vomiting, and hyperglycemia [45-47]. The isoform-selective PI3K inhibitors, currently in early phase trials in advanced solid tumors, may offer similar levels of activity in appropriately selected tumors with lower rates of adverse events.

Dual Inhibition

There are several classes of dual PI3K/AKT pathway inhibitors in clinical development. Dual mTOR/PI3K inhibitors compete for the ATP-binding sites of both mTORC complexes as well as all isoforms of PI3K. In addition, mTORC1/2 inhibitors are in development. These agents have shown promising preclinical activity *in vitro* and *in vivo*, with high sensitivity found in *PIK3CA* and *PTEN* mutant cell lines [48-52]. XL765, BEZ235, and AZD2014 are in phase I trials in advanced solid tumors, while a phase II trial of GDC-0980 in endometrial cancer is ongoing.

Potential Predictive Biomarkers for the PI3K/AKT Pathway

In the clinical experience with agents targeting the PI3K/AKT pathway, there appears to be a specific subset of women with endometrial cancer that achieve significant benefit. Despite numerous potential biomarkers, successful identification of predictive molecular profiles in endometrial cancer has been difficult. In a retrospective study, the presence of *PIK3CA* mutation in advanced solid tumors (including 3 endometrial cancers) was associated with higher than expected response to therapy (35%) with a PI3K-directed agent alone or in combination with a cytotoxic agent [53]. Retrospective evaluation of tissue in phase II trials of PI3K/AKT-targeted agents in endometrial cancer has not yielded similar results. In a study of temsirolimus as a single agent, response was independent of PTEN, phosphorylated mTOR, or phosphorylated S6K protein expression in the tumor [29]. A study of molecular determinants of response in 3 National Cancer Institute of Cancer Clinical Trials Group phase II trials of either temsirolimus or ridaforolimus yielded similar negative results. This comprehensive study explored both protein expression (PTEN or stathmin) as well as mutational status (*PIK3CA* or *PTEN*) in archival tumor specimens. No single marker or combination of markers was found to correlate with response to therapy [54]. Further, a GINECO group of 36 patients treated with everolimus found no predictor of response despite exploring expression of 10 relevant proteins and *KRAS, PIK3CA, PTEN*, and *AKT* mutation status [55]. A translational study of single agent everolimus found a trend toward correlation between presence of *KRAS* mutation and lack of response to therapy, but these results must be interpreted with caution given the small numbers and lack of power [56]. Prospective stratification by *PIK3CA* status was built into the single agent study of

MK2206 in endometrial cancer, however, there was no association between mutation status and response to therapy [41]. Interestingly, the 4 patients with clinical benefit on this trial were of serous histology [41], indicating the potential role for stratification or trial design based on histology as well as molecular profile.

RAS/RAF Pathway

Another key pathway in the development of cancer of is the RAS/RAF pathway. In addition to its functions in cell cycle survival and angiogenesis, this pathway appears to play a role in the development of resistance to targeted agents [57]. For example, the presence of *KRAS* mutation predicts failure of EGFR pathway-targeted agents in lung and colorectal cancers [58, 59]. In endometrial cancer, *KRAS* mutant cell lines are resistant to treatment with PI3K/AKT pathway-directed agents alone [60, 61]. This resistance was overcome with the addition of an agent targeting RAS/RAF in endometrial cancer cell lines with concurrent *PTEN* and *KRAS* mutation [27]. These facts, in addition to the relatively high proportion of endometrial cancers that harbor mutations in pathway members [62-64], have led to exploration of the use of agents that target the RAS/RAF pathway in this cancer type.

Targeting the RAS/RAF Pathway in Endometrial Cancer

Successfully inhibiting RAS directly has been challenging, so current efforts have focused on downstream pathway nodes, including Raf and MEK. AZD6244, a selective MEK1/2 inhibitor, was evaluated as a single agent in a phase II trial for the treatment of recurrent endometrial cancer. Six percent of patients achieved an objective response, and 26% had stable disease with this therapy [65]. Several other small molecule inhibitors of MEK are in early phase trials for advanced solid tumors. Investigators hope to improve on reported modest activity by combining these inhibitors with other targeted and cytotoxic therapies. Given the growing knowledge that *KRAS* mutations may correlate with resistance to PI3K-directed agents, the combination of AKT inhibition and MEK inhibition is under evaluation in recurrent endometrial cancer.

Potential Predictive Biomarkers for the RAS/RAF Pathway

Predictive markers have yet to be explored for MEK inhibition in endometrial cancer. However, MEK inhibition is quite developed in solid tumors such as melanoma and thyroid cancer. *BRAF* mutations have been clearly associated with response to MEK inhibition in preclinical models and clinical trials of melanoma [66, 67]. *KRAS* mutations may also correlate with response to MEK inhibition, although they do not appear to be required for response to therapy in endometrial cancer cell lines [11, 68, 69].

Angiogenesis

The growth of aberrant blood vessels within the tumor microenvironment provides increased oxygen, growth factors, and nutrients to the growing tumor. Further, angiogenesis stimulates tumor dissemination and metastasis [70, 71]. There are numerous receptors and ligands that participate in angiogenesis, including members of the vascular endothelial growth factor (VEGF) and platelet-derived growth factor (PDGF) families [72]. In addition to its impact on angiogenesis, VEGF activity may lead to proliferation, survival, and metastasis through stimulation of other transcription factors [73].

Targeting Angiogenesis in Endometrial Cancer

Expression of VEGF and other angiogenic markers has been associated with high risk tumor features and adverse outcomes in endometrial cancer [74, 75]. Indeed, preclinical studies of bevacizumab, a monoclonal antibody to VEGF-A, demonstrated an impressive reduction in tumor size in an orthotopic mouse model of endometrial cancer [74]. In endometrial cancer, targeting angiogenesis has occurred primarily through agents against VEGF-A. Bevacizumab has demonstrated the highest activity as a single agent to date. In pretreated patients, this agent achieved 2% complete response (CR), 11% PR, and 40% SD [76]. VEGF may also be targeted with afilbercept, a decoy receptor for all isoforms that binds with high affinity. A phase II trial of this agent demonstrated clinical benefit in 39% of patients with recurrent endometrial cancer [77]. In addition, sunitinib, a small molecular inhibitor of multiple VEGF receptors, has been explored in recurrent endometrial cancer. This agent achieved a response rate of 15% and 25% SD in a small phase II study [78]. These exciting results have led to additional trials of anti-angiogenic agents alone or in combination with other therapies in endometrial cancer.

Potential Predictive Biomarkers for Angiogenesis

The large number of potential markers for angiogenesis has made identification of predictive candidates challenging. Thus far, studies have been unable to correlate expression of relevant pathway members to response to anti-angiogenic therapy. For example, the expression of VEGF in serum or tissue did not correlate with response in a phase II trial of thalidomide in endometrial cancer [79]. Further, in multiple advanced solid tumors, markers such as microvessel density have failed to identify patients that will benefit from therapy [80]. Interestingly, a preclinical study of VEGF inhibition in endometrial cancer xenograft models revealed several novel markers of response and resistance which may be of interest in future clinical studies [81].

Receptor Tyrosine Kinases of Interest in Endometrial Cancer

As seen in Figure 1, the PI3K/AKT, RAS/RAF, and angiogenesis pathways may be activated by various stimuli through receptor tyrosine kinases (RTKs). Over-expression or mutation in the RTK can lead to downstream constitutive activation of the pathways, increasing tumorigenic functions within the cancer. There are numerous RTKs of importance in endometrial cancer, but targeting these aberrations has yielded little success to date. This may be secondary to difficulty in identifying molecular aberrations to predict potential responders to these agents. Of note, these agents may provide an ideal partner with PI3K-targeted agents, by reducing activation of feedback loops that stimulate continued tumorigenic functions.

Fibroblast Growth Factor Receptor 2 (FGFR2) Inhibition

Fibroblast growth factors are involved in numerous tumorigenic activities, including angiogenesis. *FGFR2* mutations are found in approximately 16% of endometrial cancers, often in the presence of loss of PTEN protein expression [12, 82]. Further, endometrial cancer cell lines with *FGFR2* mutations are sensitive to pan-FGFR inhibitors in preclinical studies [12]. Many of the agents that target FGFR also target angiogenic receptors such as VEGFR1 and VEGFR2. Results are eagerly anticipated for the trials of several FGFR inhibitors in endometrial cancer, including cedirinib, brivanib, and FP-1039. In addition, an ongoing trial of dovitinib in endometrial cancer that has employed stratification by *FGFR2* mutation status will attempt to validate a marker to predict response to this class of agents.

Insulin-like Growth Factor – 1 Receptor (IGF-IR) Inhibition

Over-expression of IGF-IR is an early molecular change in endometrial cancer and is found commonly in the precursor lesion complex atypical hyperplasia [83, 84]. The ligands of this receptor, including insulin, are quite common in obesity, a known risk factor for endometrial cancer. Further, high levels of insulin and IGF-I are associated with poor prognosis in endometrial cancer [85]. Accordingly, monoclonal antibodies to IGF-IR, ganitumab and cixutumumab, as well as the small molecular inhibitor, NVP-AEW541, have shown activity in endometrial cell lines [86-88]. Early phase trials of these agents, alone and in combination with PI3K-directed agents, are ongoing in advanced solid tumors.

Epidermal Growth Factor - 1 (EGFR) Inhibition

Inhibition of EGFR-1 (ErbB-1) has been quite successful in a variety of tumors, but this activity has not been replicated in endometrial cancer. Endometrial cancers demonstrate frequent over-expression of EGFR rather than mutation, which is rarely observed [89]. Response to EGFR therapies in lung cancer is associated with mutations, potentially explaining the disappointing results in endometrial cancer [90]. Cetuximab, a monoclonal antibody to EGFR, achieved only 5% response and 10% SD in pretreated endometrial cancer patients [91]. A small molecular inhibitor of EGFR, gefinitib, had similar low response rates [92]. Interestingly, another EGFR small molecular inhibitor, erlotinib, had improved response rates of 12% PR and 47% SD. This was likely secondary to the requirement that patients be chemonaive for inclusion [93].

Human Epidermal Growth Factor -2 (HER2) Inhibition

HER2 amplification and over-expression are more commonly found in serous compared to endometrioid endometrial tumors [17, 94]. HER2 expression is associated with poor prognosis and may predict response to chemotherapy in this disease [17, 94]. Similar to EGFR-1, activity of agents targeting HER2 has been limited. A phase II trial of trastuzumab, a monoclonal antibody, in HER2 over-expressed endometrial cancer did not achieve any objective responses although 40% of patients had SD [95] (Fleming 2010). This agent is currently under evaluation in combination with chemotherapy in advanced and recurrent uterine serous carcinoma with HER2 amplification or over-expression. A recent study has shown that a significant percentage of endometrial serous carcinomas with HER2 protein over-expression have intra-tumoral heterogeneity of *HER2* gene amplification [96]. Such heterogeneous *HER2* amplification may help to explain the limited activity of anti-HER2 targeted therapy in endometrial carcinoma. Such heterogeneous amplification is not commonly observed in breast cancers over-expressing HER2 protein [96]. Lapatinib, a dual EGFR/HER2 inhibitor, had only one response in recurrent endometrial cancer and low rates of stable disease, yielding little excitement for further development [97].

Other Targets and Agents of Interest

Estrogen

The development of endometrial cancer is known to be tightly linked to the presence of excess estrogen, especially in patients with endometrioid tumors [84]. Accordingly, hormone therapy has demonstrated moderate activity in the treatment of early and recurrent endometrioid tumors [98]. Further, estrogen signaling and the PI3K/AKT pathway interact at several levels, and hormonal resistance may occur through activation of the PI3K/AKT pathway in several tumor types [99, 100]. Targeting both pathways holds the potential for synergy in endometrial cancer. A recent phase II trial of everolimus with letrozole in pretreated endometrial cancer demonstrated significant objective response (17%, including 5 complete responses) compared to historical rates for either agent alone [101]. This combination is undergoing further evaluation in multi-center clinical trials.

Poly (ADP-Ribose) Polymerase (PARP)

Resistance to standard cytotoxic chemotherapy is found in tumors that have high activity of DNA damage repair pathways. One major avenue for DNA repair is through PARP, an enzyme that recognizes single-strand breaks within the base excision pathway. The inhibition of PARP can lead to the accumulation of double-strand breaks with subsequent cellular death after replication [102]. To avoid death, the cell can repair these double-strand breaks through the process of homologous recombination. However, if a tumor cell has an existing defect in homologous recombination, such as a mutation in *BRCA1 or BRCA2*, the DNA remains unrepaired and cell death occurs. This concept is known as synthetic lethality, and it can be seen in patients with and without *BRCA* mutations [103, 104]. For endometrial cancer, the most likely cause of homologous recombination defects is the loss of PTEN protein expression. Indeed, PARP inhibition has been shown to lead to growth inhibition in endometrial cancer cell lines [105, 106]. Studies of PARP inhibition, alone and in combination with agents that target the PI3K/AKT pathway, are ongoing in endometrial cancer.

Metformin

The biguanide agent metformin has been associated with reduced cancer risk in patients with diabetes. Further, the drug has been shown to reduce cell proliferation in a variety of different cancers, including endometrial cancer [107, 108]. Initially, the mechanism of action was thought to primarily occur through reduction of circulating insulin as well as inhibition of mTORC1 through activation of the AMP-activated protein kinase (AMPK) pathway. Recent data also reveal that metformin has its greatest impact in the inhibition of *KRAS* mutant cells. In a preclinical study by Iglesias and colleagues, metformin displaced KRAS from the membrane, thereby inhibiting its activity [109]. Thus, there are multiple potential molecular phenotypes of endometrial cancer that may benefit from this treatment. Ongoing studies are incorporating metformin into standard therapy (paclitaxel and carboplatin) as well as novel targeted therapy combinations.

Potential for Success of Targeted Therapy in Endometrial Cancer

The lack of FDA-approved agents for endometrial cancer provides a unique opportunity for the development of targeted therapy. Patients with advanced and recurrent endometrial cancer should be counseled on available options, with emphasis on participation in appropriate clinical trials. There is a clear need for exploration of targeted agents earlier in the disease process, prior to extensive pretreatment with cytotoxic chemotherapy, to reduce toxicity and maximize chance for agent success prior to the development of resistance. Further, translational objectives can be built into these trials, to allow for the identification of potential mechanisms of response and resistances. These data will inform future trial development and improve overall success. The Gynecologic Oncology Group study, GOG 86-P, is an excellent example of this strategy. This study employed a "pick the winner" design to evaluate several targeted agents (including bevacizumab, temsirolimus) in combination with paclitaxel and carboplatin.

Further, given our understanding of the extensive nature of the molecular aberrations found in endometrial cancer, the potential for success of targeted therapy in this disease is great. The majority of completed trials have focused on evaluation of these drugs as a single agent. Now that understanding exists regarding unique toxicities and considerations, we are entering the era of combination trials. This includes combination of targeted agents with standard of care chemotherapy in the upfront advanced setting, as well as the combination of cross-pathway inhibitors. These pathways employ significant feedback loops and cross talk that provide partial explanation for the modest success of targeted agents in endometrial cancer to date. Going forward, exciting combinations can be assessed based on results of prior trials and molecular characterization of this disease. Ideal combinations will include agents that address a known or proposed mechanism of resistance to a particular agent. For example, *KRAS* mutations are associated with resistance to agents targeting the PI3K/AKT pathway. Combinations that include a PI3K-directed agent and a MEK inhibitor are thought to hold great potential in endometrial cancer.

Finally, there is a huge opportunity to perform molecular analysis in endometrial cancer. At the time of primary diagnosis, there is a great deal of tissue available for assessments. Correlative studies performed prior to treatment will allow for exploration of predictive markers for outcome and response. In the recurrent setting, these patients often have highly accessible tumor for real-time assessment of markers of response during clinical trials.

Challenges to Targeted Therapy in Endometrial Cancer

Although a great deal of progress has been made in the incorporation of targeted therapy into the treatment of endometrial cancer, there are significant obstacles that exist which must be considered. Certainly, many of these issues are not unique to endometrial cancer and will need to be addressed throughout the clinical oncology community. A major challenge is development of rational clinical trial design to maximize the information generated by each study. The heterogeneous nature of the disease must be considered and addressed. For example, the molecular characteristics of endometrial cancer differ widely based on histology, which argues for separate trials by histology (endometrioid vs. non-endometrioid, for example) versus stratification within clinical trials of targeted agents. The effect of tumor histology on a specific molecular aberration are not yet known. For example, we do not know if a *PIK3CA* mutation in an endometrioid carcinoma means the same thing as a *PIK3CA* mutation in a serous carcinoma. Further, many of the trials of targeted agents have included chemonaïve and previously treated patients, limiting the conclusions that can be drawn. Thoughtful inclusion criteria are essential to the future success of targeted agents.

In general, patients with recurrent endometrial cancer typically do not undergo core needle biopsy to document metastasis. Diagnosis is often rendered using imaging or a fine need aspirate, which may limit the amount of molecular analyses that can be performed. To understand the difference in the molecular aberrations found in recurrent disease compared to primary disease, trial designs will need to incorporate pre-and post-treatment biopsies. Again, this will help to identify mechanisms for therapy resistance and guide future trial design.

Compared to many of the most common cancers, the number of patients receiving treatment for advanced and recurrent endometrial cancer is quite low. Given minimal options for standard of care treatment, these patients should be offered participation in clinical trials to increase our understanding of this disease and potentially improve patient outcomes. Further, novel trial designs, such as adaptive randomization, to maximize the information rendered by small sample size should be employed.

Conclusion

Targeted therapy is an exciting option for endometrial cancer, which is known to be one of the most molecularly aberrant solid tumors. Thus far, the success of these agents has been modest, but incorporation of novel trial design and appropriate inclusion criteria holds the potential to maximize agent success. Cross-pathway combinations and evaluation of agents earlier in the disease process holds the potential to greatly impact survival outcomes for women with this disease.

References

[1] Obel JC, Friberg G, Fleming GF. Chemotherapy in endometrial cancer. *Clin Adv Hematol Oncol.* 2006 Jun;4(6):459-68.

[2] Hanahan D, Weinberg RA. *Hallmarks of cancer: the next generation. Cell.* [Research Support, N.I.H., Extramural Review]. 2011 Mar 4;144(5):646-74.

[3] Getz G, Gabriel SB, Cibulskis K, Lander E, Sivachenko A, Sougnez C, et al. Integrated genomic characterization of endometrial carcinoma. *Nature.* 2013 May 2;497(7447):67-73.

[4] Mutter GL, Lin MC, Fitzgerald JT, Kum JB, Baak JP, Lees JA, et al. Altered PTEN expression as a diagnostic marker for the earliest endometrial precancers. *J Natl Cancer Inst.* 2000 Jun 7;92(11):924-30.

[5] Lax SF. Molecular genetic pathways in various types of endometrial carcinoma: from a phenotypical to a molecular-based classification. *Virchows Arch.* 2004 Mar;444(3):213-23.

[6] Kong D, Suzuki A, Zou TT, Sakurada A, Kemp LW, Wakatsuki S, et al. PTEN1 is frequently mutated in primary endometrial carcinomas. *Nat Genet.* 1997 Oct;17(2):143-4.

[7] Risinger JI, Hayes AK, Berchuck A, Barrett JC. PTEN/MMAC1 mutations in endometrial cancers. *Cancer Res.* 1997 Nov 1;57(21):4736-8.

[8] Velasco A, Bussaglia E, Pallares J, Dolcet X, Llobet D, Encinas M, et al. PIK3CA gene mutations in endometrial carcinoma: correlation with PTEN and K-RAS alterations. *Hum Pathol.* 2006 Nov;37(11):1465-72.

[9] Hayes MP, Wang H, Espinal-Witter R, Douglas W, Solomon GJ, Baker SJ, et al. PIK3CA and PTEN mutations in uterine endometrioid carcinoma and complex atypical hyperplasia. *Clin Cancer Res.* 2006 Oct 15;12(20 Pt 1):5932-5.

[10] Oda K, Stokoe D, Taketani Y, McCormick F. High frequency of coexistent mutations of PIK3CA and PTEN genes in endometrial carcinoma. *Cancer Res.* 2005 Dec 1;65(23):10669-73.

[11] Cheung LW, Hennessy BT, Li J, Yu S, Myers AP, Djordjevic B, et al. High Frequency of PIK3R1 and PIK3R2 Mutations in Endometrial Cancer Elucidates a Novel Mechanism for Regulation of PTEN Protein Stability. *Cancer Discov.* 2011 Jul 1;1(2):170-85.

[12] Dutt A, Salvesen HB, Chen TH, Ramos AH, Onofrio RC, Hatton C, et al. Drug-sensitive FGFR2 mutations in endometrial carcinoma. *Proc Natl Acad Sci U S A. 2008* Jun 24;105(25):8713-7.

[13] Hayes MP, Ellenson LH. Molecular alterations in uterine serous carcinoma. *Gynecol Oncol.* 2010 Feb;116(2):286-9.

[14] Lax SF, Kendall B, Tashiro H, Slebos RJ, Hedrick L. The frequency of p53, K-ras mutations, and microsatellite instability differs in uterine endometrioid and serous carcinoma: evidence of distinct molecular genetic pathways. *Cancer.* 2000 Feb 15;88(4):814-24.

[15] Schlosshauer PW, Ellenson LH, Soslow RA. Beta-catenin and E-cadherin expression patterns in high-grade endometrial carcinoma are associated with histological subtype. *Mod Pathol.* 2002 Oct;15(10):1032-7.

[16] Khalifa MA, Mannel RS, Haraway SD, Walker J, Min KW. Expression of EGFR, HER-2/neu, P53, and PCNA in endometrioid, serous papillary, and clear cell endometrial adenocarcinomas. *Gynecol Oncol.* 1994 Apr;53(1):84-92.

[17] Slomovitz BM, Broaddus RR, Burke TW, Sneige N, Soliman PT, Wu W, et al. Her-2/neu overexpression and amplification in uterine papillary serous carcinoma. *J Clin Oncol.* 2004 Aug 1;22(15):3126-32.
[18] Engelman JA, Luo J, Cantley LC. The evolution of phosphatidylinositol 3-kinases as regulators of growth and metabolism. *Nature reviews Genetics.* [Research Support, N.I.H., Extramural Review]. 2006 Aug;7(8):606-19.
[19] Meric-Bernstam F, Gonzalez-Angulo AM. Targeting the mTOR signaling network for cancer therapy. *J Clin Oncol.* 2009 May 1;27(13):2278-87.
[20] Hennessy BT, Smith DL, Ram PT, Lu Y, Mills GB. Exploiting the PI3K/AKT pathway for cancer drug discovery. *Nat Rev Drug Discov.* 2005 Dec;4(12):988-1004.
[21] Mendoza MC, Er EE, Blenis J. The Ras-ERK and PI3K-mTOR pathways: cross-talk and compensation. *Trends Biochem Sci. [Research Support, N*.I.H., Extramural Research Support, Non-U.S. Gov't Review]. 2011 Jun;36(6):320-8.
[22] Miller TW, Balko JM, Arteaga CL. Phosphatidylinositol 3-kinase and antiestrogen resistance in breast cancer. *Journal of clinical oncology : official journal of the American Society of Clinical Oncology.* [Research Support, N.I.H., Extramural Research Support, Non-U.S. Gov't Review]. 2011 Nov 20;29(33):4452-61.
[23] Whitman M, Downes CP, Keeler M, Keller T, Cantley L. Type I phosphatidylinositol kinase makes a novel inositol phospholipid, phosphatidylinositol-3-phosphate. *Nature.* [Comparative Study]. 1988 Apr 14;332(6165):644-6.
[24] Stephens L, Anderson K, Stokoe D, Erdjument-Bromage H, Painter GF, Holmes AB, et al. Protein kinase B kinases that mediate phosphatidylinositol 3,4,5-trisphosphate-dependent activation of protein kinase B. *Science.* [Research Support, Non-U.S. Gov't]. 1998 Jan 30;279(5351):710-4.
[25] Ma XM, Blenis J. Molecular mechanisms of mTOR-mediated translational control. *Nature reviews Molecular cell biology.* [Review]. 2009 May;10(5):307-18.
[26] Weigelt B, Warne PH, Lambros MB, Reis-Filho JS, Downward J, editors. Genetic determinants of mTOR inhibitor response in breast and endometrial cancer. *103rd Annual Meeting of the American Association for Cancer Research;* 2012; Chicago, IL: AACR.

[27] Shoji K, Oda K, Kashiyama T, Ikeda Y, Nakagawa S, Sone K, et al. Genotype-dependent efficacy of a dual PI3K/mTOR inhibitor, NVP-BEZ235, and an mTOR inhibitor, RAD001, in endometrial carcinomas. *PLoS One*. [Research Support, Non-U.S. Gov't]. 2012;7(5):e37431.

[28] Slomovitz BM, Lu KH, Johnston T, Coleman RL, Munsell M, Broaddus RR, et al. A phase 2 study of the oral mammalian target of rapamycin inhibitor, everolimus, in patients with recurrent endometrial carcinoma. *Cancer.* 2010 Aug 2.

[29] Oza AM, Elit L, Tsao MS, Kamel-Reid S, Biagi J, Provencher DM, et al. Phase II study of temsirolimus in women with recurrent or metastatic endometrial cancer: a trial of the NCIC Clinical Trials Group. *J Clin Oncol.* [Clinical Trial, Phase II Research Support, Non-U.S. Gov't]. 2011 Aug 20;29(24):3278-85.

[30] Oza AM, Poveda A, Clamp AR, Pignata S, Scambia G, Del Campo J, et al. A randomized phase II (RP2) trial of ridaforolimus (R) compared with progestin (P) or chemotherapy (C) in female adult patients with advanced endometrial carcinoma. *J Clin Oncol.* 2011;29 (Suppl: abstr 5009).

[31] Ray-Coquard I, Favier L, Weber B, Roemer-Becuwe C, Bougnoux P, Fabbro M, et al. Everolimus as second- or third-line treatment of advanced endometrial cancer: ENDORAD, a phase II trial of GINECO. *British journal of cancer.* [Clinical Trial, Phase II Multicenter Study Research Support, Non-U.S. Gov't]. 2013 May 14;108(9):1771-7.

[32] Colombo N, McMeekin DS, Schwartz PE, Sessa C, Gehrig PA, Holloway R, et al. Ridaforolimus as a single agent in advanced endometrial cancer: results of a single-arm, phase 2 trial. *British journal of cancer.* [Clinical Trial, Phase II Multicenter Study Research Support, Non-U.S. Gov't]. 2013 Mar 19;108(5):1021-6.

[33] Mackay H, Welch S, Tsao MS, Biagi JJ, Elit L, Ghatage P, et al. Phase II study of oral ridaforolimus in patients with metastatic and/or locally advanced recurrent endometrial cancer: NCIC CTG IND 192. *J Clin Oncol.* 2011;29 (Suppl: abstr 5013).

[34] Sarbassov DD, Guertin DA, Ali SM, Sabatini DM. Phosphorylation and regulation of Akt/PKB by the rictor-mTOR complex. *Science.* [Research Support, Non-U.S. Gov't Research Support, U.S. Gov't, P.H.S.]. 2005 Feb 18;307(5712):1098-101.

[35] West KA, Castillo SS, Dennis PA. Activation of the PI3K/Akt pathway and chemotherapeutic resistance. *Drug Resist Updat.* [Review]. 2002 Dec;5(6):234-48.

[36] Hoekstra AV, Ward EC, Hardt JL, Lurain JR, Singh DK, Buttin BM, et al. Chemosensitization of endometrial cancer cells through AKT inhibition involves FOXO1. *Gynecologic oncology.* [Research Support, Non-U.S. Gov't]. 2008 Mar;108(3):609-18.

[37] Gagnon V, Mathieu I, Sexton E, Leblanc K, Asselin E. AKT involvement in cisplatin chemoresistance of human uterine cancer cells. *Gynecologic oncology.* [Research Support, Non-U.S. Gov't]. 2004 Sep;94(3):785-95.

[38] Chandarlapaty S, Sawai A, Scaltriti M, Rodrik-Outmezguine V, Grbovic-Huezo O, Serra V, et al. AKT inhibition relieves feedback suppression of receptor tyrosine kinase expression and activity. *Cancer Cell.* [Research Support, N.I.H., Extramural]. 2011 Jan 18;19(1):58-71.

[39] Block M, Fister S, Emons G, Seeber S, Grundker C, Gunthert AR. Antiproliferative effects of antiestrogens and inhibitors of growth factor receptor signaling on endometrial cancer cells. *Anticancer Res.* [Research Support, Non-U.S. Gov't]. 2010 Jun;30(6):2025-31.

[40] Hirai H, Sootome H, Nakatsuru Y, Miyama K, Taguchi S, Tsujioka K, et al. MK-2206, an allosteric Akt inhibitor, enhances antitumor efficacy by standard chemotherapeutic agents or molecular targeted drugs in vitro and in vivo. *Mol Cancer Ther.* [Research Support, Non-U.S. Gov't]. 2010 Jul;9(7):1956-67.

[41] Myers AP, Broaddus R, Makker V, Konstantinopoulos P, Drapkin R, Horowitz NS, et al. Phase II, two-stage, two-arm, PIK3CA mutation stratified trial of MK-2206 in recurrent endometrial cancer. *J Clin Oncol.* 2013;31 (suppl; abstr 5524).

[42] Maira SM, Pecchi S, Huang A, Burger M, Knapp M, Sterker D, et al. Identification and characterization of NVP-BKM120, an orally available pan-class I PI3-kinase inhibitor. *Mol Cancer Ther.* 2012 Feb;11(2):317-28.

[43] Folkes AJ, Ahmadi K, Alderton WK, Alix S, Baker SJ, Box G, et al. The identification of 2-(1H-indazol-4-yl)-6-(4-methanesulfonyl-piperazin-1-ylmethyl)-4-morpholin-4-yl-t hieno[3,2-d]pyrimidine (GDC-0941) as a potent, selective, orally bioavailable inhibitor of class I PI3 kinase for the treatment of cancer. *J Med Chem.* 2008 Sep 25;51(18):5522-32.

[44] Sos ML, Fischer S, Ullrich R, Peifer M, Heuckmann JM, Koker M, et al. Identifying genotype-dependent efficacy of single and combined PI3K- and MAPK-pathway inhibition in cancer. *Proc Natl Acad Sci U S* A. [Research Support, N.I.H., Extramural Research Support, Non-U.S. Gov't]. 2009 Oct 27;106(43):18351-6.

[45] Bendell JC, Rodon J, Burris HA, de Jonge M, Verweij J, Birle D, et al. Phase I, dose-escalation study of BKM120, an oral pan-Class I PI3K inhibitor, in patients with advanced solid tumors. *J Clin Oncol.* [Clinical Trial, Phase I Research Support, Non-U.S. Gov't]. 2012 Jan 20;30(3):282-90.

[46] Edelman G, Bedell C, Sharpiro G, Pandya SS, Kwak EL, Scheffold C, et al. A phase I dose-escalation study of XL 147 (SAR245408), a PI3K inhibitor adminstered orally to patients (pts) with advanced malignancies. *J Clin Oncol.* 2010;28: 15s (suppl; abstr 3004).

[47] Von Hoff DD, LoRusso P, Demetri GD, Weiss GJ, Shapiro G, Ramanathan RK, et al. A phase I dose-escalation study to evaluate GDC-0941, a pan-PI3K inhibitor, administered QD to BID in advanced or metastatic solid tumors. *J Clin Oncol.* 2011;29 (suppl; abstr 3052).

[48] Wallin JJ, Edgar KA, Guan J, Berry M, Prior WW, Lee L, et al. GDC-0980 is a novel class I PI3K/mTOR kinase inhibitor with robust activity in cancer models driven by the PI3K pathway. *Mol Cancer Ther.* 2011 Dec;10(12):2426-36.

[49] Maira SM, Stauffer F, Brueggen J, Furet P, Schnell C, Fritsch C, et al. Identification and characterization of NVP-BEZ235, a new orally available dual phosphatidylinositol 3-kinase/mammalian target of rapamycin inhibitor with potent in vivo antitumor activity. *Mol Cancer Ther.* 2008 Jul;7(7):1851-63.

[50] Chresta CM, Davies BR, Hickson I, Harding T, Cosulich S, Critchlow SE, et al. AZD8055 is a potent, selective, and orally bioavailable ATP-competitive mammalian target of rapamycin kinase inhibitor with in vitro and in vivo antitumor activity. *Cancer Res.* 2010 Jan 1;70(1):288-98.

[51] Korets SB, Musa F, Curtin J, Blank SV, Schneider RJ. Dual mTORC1/2 inhibition in a preclinical xenograft tumor model of endometrial cancer. *Gynecol Oncol.* 2013 Dec 4.

[52] Pike KG, Malagu K, Hummersone MG, Menear KA, Duggan HM, Gomez S, et al. Optimization of potent and selective dual mTORC1 and mTORC2 inhibitors: the discovery of AZD8055 and AZD2014. *Bioorganic & medicinal chemistry letters.* 2013 Mar 1;23(5):1212-6.

[53] Janku F, Tsimberidou AM, Garrido-Laguna I, Wang X, Luthra R, Hong DS, et al. PIK3CA mutations in patients with advanced cancers treated with PI3K/AKT/mTOR axis inhibitors. *Mol Cancer Ther.* 2011 Mar;10(3):558-65.

[54] Mackay HJ, Eisenhauer EA, Kamel-Reid S, Tsao M, Clarke B, Karakasis K, et al. Molecular determinants of outcome with mammalian target of rapamycin inhibition in endometrial cancer. *Cancer.* 2013 Oct 25.

[55] Tredan O, Treilleux I, Wang Q, Gane N, Pissaloux D, Bonnin N, et al. Predicting everolimus treatment efficacy in patients with advanced endometrial carcinoma: a GINECO group study. *Target Oncol.* 2013 Dec;8(4):243-51.

[56] Meyer LA, Slomovitz BM, Djordjevic B, Galbincea JM, Johnston TA, Munsell M, et al. The search continues: looking for predictive biomarkers for response mTOR inhibition in endometrial cancer. *J Clin Oncol.* 2011;29 (Suppl; abstr 5016).

[57] Montagut C, Settleman J. Targeting the RAF-MEK-ERK pathway in cancer therapy. *Cancer Lett.* 2009 Oct 8;283(2):125-34.

[58] Massarelli E, Varella-Garcia M, Tang X, Xavier AC, Ozburn NC, Liu DD, et al. KRAS mutation is an important predictor of resistance to therapy with epidermal growth factor receptor tyrosine kinase inhibitors in non-small-cell lung cancer. *Clin Cancer Res.* 2007 May 15;13(10):2890-6.

[59] Jimeno A, Messersmith WA, Hirsch FR, Franklin WA, Eckhardt SG. KRAS mutations and sensitivity to epidermal growth factor receptor inhibitors in colorectal cancer: practical application of patient selection. *J Clin Oncol.* 2009 Mar 1;27(7):1130-6.

[60] Engelman JA, Chen L, Tan X, Crosby K, Guimaraes AR, Upadhyay R, et al. Effective use of PI3K and MEK inhibitors to treat mutant Kras G12D and PIK3CA H1047R murine lung cancers. *Nat Med.* 2008 Dec;14(12):1351-6.

[61] Ihle NT, Lemos R, Jr., Wipf P, Yacoub A, Mitchell C, Siwak D, et al. Mutations in the phosphatidylinositol-3-kinase pathway predict for antitumor activity of the inhibitor PX-866 whereas oncogenic Ras is a dominant predictor for resistance. *Cancer Res.* [Research Support, N.I.H., Extramural]. 2009 Jan 1;69(1):143-50.

[62] Samarnthai N, Hall K, Yeh IT. Molecular profiling of endometrial malignancies. *Obstetrics and gynecology international.* 2010;2010:162363.

[63] Varras MN, Koffa M, Koumantakis E, Ergazaki M, Protopapa E, Michalas S, et al. ras gene mutations in human endometrial carcinoma. *Oncology.* 1996 Nov-Dec;53(6):505-10.

[64] Koul A, Willen R, Bendahl PO, Nilbert M, Borg A. Distinct sets of gene alterations in endometrial carcinoma implicate alternate modes of tumorigenesis. *Cancer.* 2002 May 1;94(9):2369-79.

[65] Coleman R, Sill M, Thaker PH, De Geest K, Street D, McGuire W, et al. A phase II evaluation of AZD6244, a selective MEK-1/2 inhibitor in the treatment of recurrent or persistent endometrial cancer: A Gynecologic Oncology Group study. *Gynecol Oncol.* 2013;130(1):e12-3.

[66] Dummer R, Robert C, Chapman PB, Sosman JA, Middleton M, Bastholt L, et al. AZD6244 (ARRY-142886) vs temozolomide (TMZ) in patients (pts) with advanced melanoma: An open-label, randomized, multicenter, phase II study. *J Clin Oncol.* 2008;26: Suppl; abstr 9033.

[67] Patel SP, Lazar AJ, Mahoney S, Vaughn C, Gonzalez N, Papadopoulos NE, et al., editors. *Clinical responses to AZD6244 (ARRY-142886)-based combination therapy stratified by gene mutations in patients with metastatic melanoma.* 2010 ASCO Molecular Markers; 2010.

[68] Friday BB, Adjei AA. Advances in targeting the Ras/Raf/MEK/Erk mitogen-activated protein kinase cascade with MEK inhibitors for cancer therapy. *Clin Cancer Res.* 2008 Jan 15;14(2):342-6.

[69] Chapman MS, Miner JN. Novel mitogen-activated protein kinase kinase inhibitors. Expert Opin Investig Drugs. 2011 Feb;20(2):209-20.

[70] Folkman J. What is the evidence that tumors are angiogenesis dependent? *J Natl Cancer Inst.* 1990 Jan 3;82(1):4-6.

[71] Hicklin DJ, Ellis LM. Role of the vascular endothelial growth factor pathway in tumor growth and angiogenesis. *J Clin Oncol.* 2005 Feb 10;23(5):1011-27.

[72] Samples J, Willis M, Klauber-Demore N. Targeting angiogenesis and the tumor microenvironment. *Surg Oncol Clin N Am.* 2013 Oct;22(4):629-39.

[73] Ellis LM, Hicklin DJ. VEGF-targeted therapy: mechanisms of anti-tumour activity. *Nature reviews Cancer.* [Review]. 2008 Aug;8(8):579-91.

[74] Kamat AA, Merritt WM, Coffey D, Lin YG, Patel PR, Broaddus R, et al. Clinical and biological significance of vascular endothelial growth factor in endometrial cancer. *Clin Cancer Res.* 2007 Dec 15;13(24):7487-95.

[75] Stefansson IM, Salvesen HB, Akslen LA. Vascular proliferation is important for clinical progress of endometrial cancer. *Cancer research.* [Research Support, Non-U.S. Gov't]. 2006 Mar 15;66(6):3303-9.

[76] Aghajanian C, Sill MW, Darcy K, Greer B, McMeekin DS, Rose PG, et al. A phase II evaluation of bevacizumab in the treatment of recurrent or

persistant endometrial cancer: *A Gynecologic Oncology Group* (GOG) study. J Clin Oncol. 2009;27:15s (suppl; abstr 5531).

[77] Coleman RL, Sill MW, Lankes HA, Fader AN, Finkler NJ, Hoffman JS, et al. A phase II evaluation of aflibercept in the treatment of recurrent or persistent endometrial cancer: a Gynecologic Oncology Group study. *Gynecologic oncology.* [Clinical Trial, Phase II Research Support, N.I.H., Extramural Research Support, Non-U.S. Gov't]. 2012 Dec;127(3):538-43.

[78] Correa R, Mackay H, Hirte HW, Morgan R, Welch S, Fleming GF, et al. A phase II study of sunitinib in recurrent or metastastic endometrial carcinoma: A trial of the Princess Margaret Hospital, The University of Chicago, and California Cancer Phase II Consortia. *J Clin Oncol.* 2010;28: 15s (suppl; abstr 5038).

[79] McMeekin DS, Sill MW, Benbrook D, Darcy KM, Stearns-Kurosawa DJ, Eaton L, et al. A phase II trial of thalidomide in patients with refractory endometrial cancer and correlation with angiogenesis biomarkers: a Gynecologic Oncology Group study. *Gynecol Oncol.* 2007 May;105(2):508-16.

[80] Jubb AM, Harris AL. Biomarkers to predict the clinical efficacy of bevacizumab in cancer. *The lancet oncology.* [Research Support, Non-U.S. Gov't Review]. 2010 Dec;11(12):1172-83.

[81] Davies S, Dai D, Pickett G, Thiel KW, Korovkina VP, Leslie KK. Effects of bevacizumab in mouse model of endometrial cancer: Defining the molecular basis for resistance. *Oncology reports.* [Research Support, N.I.H., *Extramural Research Support,* Non-U.S. Gov't]. 2011 Mar;25(3):855-62.

[82] Byron SA, Gartside MG, Wellens CL, Mallon MA, Keenan JB, Powell MA, et al. Inhibition of activated fibroblast growth factor receptor 2 in endometrial cancer cells induces cell death despite PTEN abrogation. *Cancer Res.* 2008 Sep 1;68(17):6902-7.

[83] McCampbell AS, Broaddus RR, Loose DS, Davies PJ. Overexpression of the insulin-like growth factor I receptor and activation of the AKT pathway in hyperplastic endometrium. *Clin Cancer Res.* 2006 Nov 1;12(21):6373-8.

[84] Westin SN, Broaddus RR, Deng L, McCampbell A, Lu KH, Lacour RA, et al. Molecular clustering of endometrial carcinoma based on estrogen-induced gene expression. *Cancer Biol Ther.* 2009 Nov;8(22):2126-35.

[85] Gallagher EJ, LeRoith D. Minireview: IGF, Insulin, and Cancer. *Endocrinology.* [Review]. 2011 Jul;152(7):2546-51.

[86] Attias-Geva Z, Bentov I, Fishman A, Werner H, Bruchim I. Insulin-like growth factor-I receptor inhibition by specific tyrosine kinase inhibitor NVP-AEW541 in endometrioid and serous papillary endometrial cancer cell lines. *Gynecol Oncol.* 2011 May 1;121(2):383-9.

[87] Mendivil A, Zhou C, Cantrell LA, Gehrig PA, Malloy KM, Blok LJ, et al. AMG 479, a novel IGF-1-R antibody, inhibits endometrial cancer cell proliferation through disruption of the PI3K/Akt and MAPK pathways. *Reprod Sci.* [Research Support, N.I.H., Extramural Research Support, Non-U.S. Gov't]. 2011 Sep;18(9):832-41.

[88] Attias-Geva Z, Bentov I, Ludwig DL, Fishman A, Bruchim I, Werner H. Insulin-like growth factor-I receptor (IGF-IR) targeting with monoclonal antibody cixutumumab (IMC-A12) inhibits IGF-I action in endometrial cancer cells. *European journal of cancer.* [Research Support, Non-U.S. Gov't]. 2011 Jul;47(11):1717-26.

[89] Pfeiffer D, Spranger J, Al-Deiri M, Kimmig R, Fisseler-Eckhoff A, Scheidel P, et al. mRNA expression of ligands of the epidermal-growth-factor-receptor in the uterus. *International journal of cancer Journal international du cancer.* [Research Support, Non-U.S. Gov't]. 1997 Aug 7;72(4):581-6.

[90] Langer CJ. *Roles of EGFR and KRAS Mutations in the Treatment Of Patients With Non-Small-Cell Lung Cancer.* P T. 2011 May;36(5):263-79.

[91] Slomovitz BM, Schmeler K, Miller DS, Lu K, Ramirez PT, Caputo T, et al. Phase II study of cetuximab (Erbitux) in patients with progressive or recurrent endometrial cancer. *Gynecol Oncol.* 2010;166 (suppl; abstr 13).

[92] Leslie KK, Sill MW, Darcy KM, Baron AT, Wilken JA, Godwin AK, et al. Efficacy and safety of gefitinib and potential prognostic value of soluble EGFR, EGFR mutations, and tumor markers in a Gynecologic Oncology Group phase II trial of persistent or recurrent endometrial cancer. *J Clin Oncol.* 2009;27 (Suppl: abstr e16542).

[93] Oza AM, Eisenhauer EA, Elit L, Cutz JC, Sakurada A, Tsao MS, et al. Phase II study of erlotinib in recurrent or metastatic endometrial cancer: NCIC IND-148. *J Clin Oncol.* 2008 Sep 10;26(26):4319-25.

[94] Santin AD, Bellone S, Gokden M, Palmieri M, Dunn D, Agha J, et al. Overexpression of HER-2/neu in uterine serous papillary cancer. *Clin Cancer Res.* 2002 May;8(5):1271-9.

[95] Fleming GF, Sill MW, Darcy KM, McMeekin DS, Thigpen JT, Adler LM, et al. Phase II trial of trastuzumab in women with advanced or

recurrent, HER2-positive endometrial carcinoma: a Gynecologic Oncology Group study. *Gynecol Oncol.* 2009 Jan;116(1):15-20.

[96] Buza N, Hui P. Marked heterogeneity of HER2/NEU gene amplification in endometrial serous carcinoma. *Genes, chromosomes & cancer.* 2013 Oct 7.

[97] Leslie KK, Sill MW, Lankes HA, Fischer EG, Godwin AK, Gray H, et al. Lapatinib and potential prognostic value of EGFR mutations in a Gynecologic Oncology Group phase II trial of persistent or recurrent endometrial cancer. *Gynecologic oncology.* [Clinical Trial, Phase II Multicenter Study Research Support, N.I.H., Extramural Research Support, Non-U.S. Gov't]. 2012 Nov;127(2):345-50.

[98] Gunderson CC, Fader AN, Carson KA, Bristow RE. Oncologic and reproductive outcomes with progestin therapy in women with endometrial hyperplasia and grade 1 adenocarcinoma: a systematic review. *Gynecol Oncol.* [Research Support, N.I.H., Extramural Research Support, Non-U.S. Gov't Review]. 2012 May;125(2):477-82.

[99] Zhang Z, Dong L, Sui L, Yang Y, Liu X, Yu Y, et al. Metformin reverses progestin resistance in endometrial cancer cells by downregulating GloI expression. I*nt J Gynecol Cancer.* 2011 Feb;21(2):213-21.

[100] Gu C, Zhang Z, Yu Y, Liu Y, Zhao F, Yin L, et al. Inhibiting the PI3K/Akt pathway reversed progestin resistance in endometrial cancer. *Cancer science.* [Research Support, Non-U.S. Gov't]. 2011 Mar;102(3):557-64.

[101] Slomovitz BM, Brown J, Johnston TA, Mura D, Levenback C, Wolf J, et al. A phase II study of everolimus and letrozole in patients with recurrent endometrial cancer. *J Clin Oncol.* 2011;29 (Suppl: abstr 5012).

[102] Gien LT, Mackay HJ. The Emerging Role of PARP Inhibitors in the Treatment of Epithelial Ovarian Cancer. *J Oncol.* 2010:ID 151750.

[103] Dedes KJ, Wilkerson PM, Wetterskog D, Weigelt B, Ashworth A, Reis-Filho JS. Synthetic lethality of PARP inhibition in cancers lacking BRCA1 and BRCA2 mutations. Cell Cycle. 2011 Apr 15;10(8):1192-9.

[104] Fong PC, Boss DS, Yap TA, Tutt A, Wu P, Mergui-Roelvink M, et al. Inhibition of poly(ADP-ribose) polymerase in tumors from BRCA mutation carriers. *N Engl J Med.* 2009 Jul 9;361(2):123-34.

[105] Dedes KJ, Wetterskog D, Mendes-Pereira AM, Natrajan R, Lambros MB, Geyer FC, et al. PTEN deficiency in endometrioid endometrial adenocarcinomas predicts sensitivity to PARP inhibitors. *Sci Transl Med.* 2010 Oct 13;2(53):53ra75.

[106] Mendes-Pereira AM, Martin SA, Brough R, McCarthy A, Taylor JR, Kim JS, et al. Synthetic lethal targeting of PTEN mutant cells with PARP inhibitors. *EMBO Mol Med.* 2009 Sep;1(6-7):315-22.

[107] Li D. Metformin as an Antitumor Agent in Cancer Prevention and Treatment. *J Diabetes.* 2011 Feb 21.

[108] Dowling RJ, Goodwin PJ, Stambolic V. Understanding the benefit of metformin use in cancer treatment. *BMC Med.* [Research Support, Non-U.S. Gov't Review]. 2011;9:33.

[109] Iglesias DA, Yates MS, van der Hoeven D, Rodkey TL, Zhang Q, Co NN, et al. Another Surprise from Metformin: Novel Mechanism of Action via K-Ras Influences Endometrial Cancer Response to Therapy. *Molecular cancer therapeutics.* 2013 Dec;12(12):2847-56.

[110] Djordjevic B, Hennessy BT, Li J, Barkoh BA, Luthra R, Mills GB, et al. Clinical assessment of PTEN loss in endometrial carcinoma: immunohistochemistry outperforms gene sequencing. *Mod Pathol.* [Comparative StudyResearch Support, N.I.H., Extramural Research Support, Non-U.S. Gov't]. 2012 May;25(5):699-708.

[111] Urick ME, Rudd ML, Godwin AK, Sgroi D, Merino M, Bell DW. PIK3R1 (p85alpha) is somatically mutated at high frequency in primary endometrial cancer. *Cancer Res.* 2011 Jun 15;71(12):4061-7.

[112] Dutt A, Salvesen HB, Greulich H, Sellers WR, Beroukhim R, Meyerson M. Somatic mutations are present in all members of the AKT family in endometrial carcinoma. *Br J Cancer.* 2009 Oct 6;101(7):1218-9; author reply 20-1.

[113] Shoji K, Oda K, Nakagawa S, Hosokawa S, Nagae G, Uehara Y, et al. The oncogenic mutation in the pleckstrin homology domain of AKT1 in endometrial carcinomas. *Br J Cancer.* 2009 Jul 7;101(1):145-8.

[114] Pollock PM, Gartside MG, Dejeza LC, Powell MA, Mallon MA, Davies H, et al. Frequent activating FGFR2 mutations in endometrial carcinomas parallel germline mutations associated with craniosynostosis and skeletal dysplasia syndromes. *Oncogene.* 2007 Nov 1;26(50):7158-62.

[115] Bigsby RM, Li AX, Bomalaski J, Stehman FB, Look KY, Sutton GP. Immunohistochemical study of HER-2/neu, epidermal growth factor receptor, and steroid receptor expression in normal and malignant endometrium. *Obstet Gynecol.* 1992 Jan;79(1):95-100.

[116] Grushko TA, Filiaci VL, Mundt AJ, Ridderstrale K, Olopade OI, Fleming GF. An exploratory analysis of HER-2 amplification and

overexpression in advanced endometrial carcinoma: a Gynecologic Oncology Group study. *Gynecol Oncol.* 2008 Jan;108(1):3-9.

[117] Schlosshauer PW, Pirog EC, Levine RL, Ellenson LH. Mutational analysis of the CTNNB1 and APC genes in uterine endometrioid carcinoma. *Mod Pathol.* 2000 Oct;13(10):1066-71.

[118] Ragni N, Ferrero S, Prefumo F, Muschiato B, Gorlero F, Gualco M, et al. The association between p53 expression, stage and histological features in endometrial cancer. *European journal of obstetrics, gynecology, and reproductive biology.* 2005 Nov 1;123(1):111-6.

[119] Zannoni GF, Vellone VG, Arena V, Prisco MG, Scambia G, Carbone A, et al. Does high-grade endometrioid carcinoma (grade 3 FIGO) belong to type I or type II endometrial cancer? A clinical-pathological and immunohistochemical study. *Virchows Arch.* 2010 Jul;457(1):27-34.

[120] Moreno-Bueno G, Hardisson D, Sarrio D, Sanchez C, Cassia R, Prat J, et al. Abnormalities of E- and P-cadherin and catenin (beta-, gamma-catenin, and p120ctn) expression in endometrial cancer and endometrial atypical hyperplasia. *J Pathol.* 2003 Apr;199(4):471-8.

[121] Holcomb K, Delatorre R, Pedemonte B, McLeod C, Anderson L, Chambers J. E-cadherin expression in endometrioid, papillary serous, and clear cell carcinoma of the endometrium. *Obstet Gynecol.* 2002 Dec;100(6):1290-5.

[122] MacDonald ND, Salvesen HB, Ryan A, Iversen OE, Akslen LA, Jacobs IJ. Frequency and prognostic impact of microsatellite instability in a large population-based study of endometrial carcinomas. *Cancer Res.* 2000 Mar 15;60(6):1750-2.

[123] Basil JB, Goodfellow PJ, Rader JS, Mutch DG, Herzog TJ. Clinical significance of microsatellite instability in endometrial carcinoma. *Cancer.* 2000 Oct 15;89(8):1758-64.

[124] Hayes MP, Douglas W, Ellenson LH. Molecular alterations of EGFR and PIK3CA in uterine serous carcinoma. *Gynecol Oncol.* 2009 Jun;113(3):370-3.

[125] Soong R, Knowles S, Hammond IG, Michael C, Iacopetta BJ. p53 protein overexpression and gene mutation in mixed Mullerian tumors of the uterus. *Cancer detection and prevention.* 1999;23(1):8-12.

Editors' Contact Information

Dr. Ivan Diaz-Padilla
Consultant Medical Oncologist
Gynecologic Cancer Program
Division of Medical Oncology
Centro Intergral Oncologico Clara Campal
University Hospital HM Madrid
10 Oña; 28050 Sanchinarro; Madrid, Spain
Tel: (+34) 91-756-78-00
Fax: (+34) 91-750-79-31
E-mail: ivandpadilla@hospitaldemadrid.com

Dr. Jesus Garcia-Donas
Consultant Medical Oncologist
Gynecologic Cancer Program
Division of Medical Oncology
Centro Intergral Oncologico Clara Campal
University Hospital HM Madrid
10 Oña; 28050 Sanchinarro; Madrid, Spain
Tel: (+34) 91-756-78-00
Fax: (+34) 91-750-79-31
E-mail:jgarciadonas@gmail.com

Index

B

C

D

E

F

G

H

I

J

K

L

M

N

O

P

Q

R

S

T